INTERMITTENT FASTING 16/8

The Essential Beginner's Guide
with the 16/8 Method.
How to Heal your Body
and Live a Healthy Lifestyle

ALICIA LYNN

CONTENTS

INTRODUCTION

Over half of the world's population is overweight. Think about it for a moment: it's worrisome how quickly the incidence of obesity and overweight has increased in the past 30 years. This growing trend of overweight people has prompted the food and supplement industry to use it as an opportunity to make billions of profits, often promoting products that have no value and are ineffective when it comes to losing excess fat body. Although there are so many diet programs and pills on the market that are not supported by scientific research or evidence that often lead to unwanted results, all is not lost. Some strategies have proven effective in long-term weight loss. By following a well-planned approach, you can safely lose weight (losing weight too quickly is harmful), and you can maintain it for many years, provided it leads to a healthy lifestyle and follows your habits. One special strategy that has become popular with people who want to lead healthier lives and lose weight at the same time is intermittent fasting. Intermittent fasting has long been a hunger technique and therefore has a relatively small feeding window where all meals during the day need to be regulated. Although scientific studies have shown that intermittent fasting is a useful tool for losing weight, it should also be taken into account that if there is no adequately planned strategy, no diet program focused on weight loss will produce results that can be an achievement.

However, if you are not sure how to start, where to start, when to eat, what program to follow, and of course, what to eat, don't worry. This book will find a complete guide on what you should eat, how to calculate the desired calorie intake, and how much you should eat. I will also share the most important reasons why an intermittent fasting diet plays a key role in keeping your body in good shape and health. For those who don't know much about intermittent fasting, except that it has helped many people lose weight, I will start this book with a general overview of intermittent fasting in general, as well as specific intermittent fasting. I'll also give you a brief description of how to determine what you should eat based on your purpose and give you an overview of the various options you can choose when preparing meals (which, incidentally, are delicious).

.

CHAPTER 1 - SOCIAL PHENOMENON OF OBESITY

Let's quickly start looking into the causes of the increase in body weight and obesity.

The cortisol

The repeated rise of cortisol can lead to weight gain. Cortisol can mobilize triglycerides from the bed and transfer them to the visceral fat cells (located under the muscles, deep in the abdomen). Cortisol also helps in the development of adipocytes in mature fat cells. The biochemical process at the cellular level concerns the enzymatic control (dehydrogenase), which converts cortisone into cortisol in adipose tissue. Higher numbers of these enzymes in visceral fat cells can lead to increased cortisol production at the tissue level, causing injury (because the adrenal glands are already pumping cortisol). Also, physical fat cells have more cortisol receptors than subcutaneous fat.

The second way cortisol can participate in weight gain has to do with the blood sugar problem. Consistently high blood glucose levels associated with insulin suppression lead to glucose deficient cells. But these cells are asking for energy, and one way of regulation is to send hunger signals to the brain. This can lead to overeating. And of course, unused glucose is eventually stored as fat.

Another combination is the effect of cortisol on appetite and the hunger for high-calorie foods. Studies have shown a direct relationship between cortisol levels and calorie intake in female populations. It can directly affect thirst and appetite by binding to hypothalamus receptors in the brain. Cortisol also indirectly affects appetite by modulating other hormones and stress-sensitive factors known to stimulate the appetite.

Suppression of the immune system

Cortisol works to reduce inflammation in the body, which is positive, but over time these efforts to reduce inflammation also suppress the immune system. Chronic inflammation caused by lifestyle factors such as poor nutrition and stress helps maintain cortisol levels, causing chaos in the immune system. An uncontrolled immune system that responds to weakened inflammation can lead to countless problems: increased susceptibility to colds and other diseases, increased risk of cancer, the tendency to food allergies, increased risk of various gastrointestinal problems and probably an increased risk of autoimmune diseases.

Nervous system

Cortisol activates the sympathetic nervous system, causing all the physiological reactions described above. The parasympathetic nervous system has to be suppressed because both systems cannot function simultaneously. The parasympathetic nervous system is stimulated during silent activities such as food, which is essential because, for better use of food energy, the enzymes and hormones that control digestion and absorption must function at maximum efficiency.

Imagine what happens in the stressful and flooded cortisol while you eat: digestion and absorption are compromised, indigestion develops, and the mucous membrane becomes irritated and inflamed. This may seem familiar. Ulcers are more common in stressful times, and many people with irritable bowel syndrome and colitis report improved symptoms when they dominate stress management.

Of course, the resulting mucosa's inflammation leads to an increase in cortisol production, and the cycle continues as the body becomes increasingly stressed.

Cardiovascular disease

As we have seen, cortisol compresses blood vessels and increases blood pressure to improve oxygenated blood supply. This is useful in combat or flight situations, but not always. Over time, such a narrowing of the arteries and high blood pressure can cause vascular damage and plaque buildup, which is an ideal scenario for a heart attack.

Fertility issues

High cortisol levels associated with prolonged stress can lead to erectile dysfunction or normal ovulation and menstrual cycles. Also, androgen sex hormones are produced in the same glands as cortisol and epinephrine, so excessive cortisol production can hinder the optimal production of these sex hormones.

Other problems.

Prolonged stress and high cortisol levels can also be associated with insomnia, chronic fatigue syndrome, thyroid disorders, dementia, depression, and other conditions.

Cortisol Evaluation

Adrenal Stress Index (ASI), the salivary test, is the preferred test for adrenal function and a reliable, non-invasive, and well-accepted indicator of cortisol levels. A qualified specialist should interpret the results because of factors such as age, sex, time with the menstrual cycle, pregnancy, breastfeeding, smoking, medications, medical conditions, intake of caffeine and alcohol, calorie intake and other test results. ASI is available as a home kit: four saliva samples are taken at specific times and then sent to the laboratory for analysis. Conveniently, in addition to measuring adrenal hormones, cortisol, and dehydroepiandrosterone, the same test also measures gliadin antibodies, often used as a marker of enteritis, candida infection and gluten-sensitive cereals.

A blood cortisol test is available, but it is considered inferior to a salivary test for three reasons: it tests cortisol levels only at a given time, which provides information four times lower than the levels (which reveals significant imbalances); A blood test alone (or simply going to the doctor) can stress a person enough to cause an increase in cortisol levels, and is considered less sensitive because it measures total hormone levels compared to specific ingredients.

The good news

So far, it may seem that stressed people are doomed, and not to be able to live despite their best intentions. Fortunately, there is much we can do for ourselves to reverse the path of destruction. The best way to avoid cortisol is to master stress management and optimize your diet.

Stress management

First, regardless of the scope of our practice, we can always recommend strategies for effective stress management. Books such as source Woodson Merrell, have a powerful suggestion, but guided by common sense, based on testing stress conditions and regaining optimal health. Some strategies include improving sleep quality, breathing, acupuncture, cardio/resistance/relaxation exercises, and solving psychological/emotional problems.

Anti-inflammatory diet.

Systemic inflammation, as mentioned above, causes high levels of cortisol. If we can naturally reduce inflammation in the body and minimize stress, they should follow a reduced cortisol level, resulting in a lower risk of chronic diseases and better health. The biochemical processes that bring and reduce inflammation are complex and multifaceted, but as diet and lifestyle experts, we can make a significant difference.

Like any diet designed to control the condition, there is no perfect anti-inflammatory diet. However, according to the food properties and known clinical studies, we can design a low inflammation diet in general and adapt it over time. Of course, maximizing anti-inflammatory effects and minimizing anti-inflammatory effects is a big step in controlling inflammation. By the way, dietary strategies for controlling inflammation can also generally help maintain the adrenal glands, because diet can directly affect the load of the adrenal glands (for example, cortisol is released in response to metabolic needs).

Since lifestyle is usually the most important modulators of inflammation, diet can have a big impact on the general condition of ourselves. Below is a general list of factors considered in the diet and lifestyle that contribute to inflammation:

- High glycemic load;
- Saturated and trans fatty acids;
- Caffeine;
- Excess alcohol;
- Insufficient intake of microelements and antioxidants;
- The diet is low in fiber;
- A sedentary lifestyle

To minimize inflammation, we recommend:

- Low glycemic load diet;
- Elimination of Tran's fats and minimal consumption of saturated fats;
- Elimination or reduction of caffeine;
- Alcohol in moderation or not at all;
- Increase the food intake of whole plants to maximize the intake of fiber, antioxidants, and nutrients: with vegetables, fruit, intact whole grains, nuts, seeds, and beans;

• Meet the recommended intake of omega-3 fatty acids (better measured as the proportion of omega-6 fatty acids);

• Regular exercise;

• Probiotics, if justified.

Of course, these are only guidelines. Therapeutic recommendations on nutrition should be tailored to each person's conditions, preferences, and goals.

Bear in mind that although drugs such as NSAIDs temporarily relieve inflammation, hundreds of studies have shown that long-term use can cause harm over time, and even systemic inflammation exacerbates.

Cortisol is a fascinating hormone that is important for learning about nutrition on many levels. Understanding the science that supports it, including its behavior and relationships with other biochemical components, the immune system, and health outcomes, is critical to our success in treating people seeking dietary intervention for stress, disease, fatigue, and other common conditions.

The implementation of specific nutrition and lifestyle methods is an extremely effective way to reduce stress, minimize inflammation, and reduce the risk of diseases and chronic diseases. Indeed, many biochemical processes, including cortisol and other hormones, stress, and inflammation, as well as their impact on health and disease risk, are complex and complicated. However, therapeutic diets and lifestyle strategies are not. The more we learn about how the body meets the requirements, as well as its extraordinary healing power, the more we appreciate ourselves as professionals who can change people's lives, improve health, inspire change and extend life.

CORTISOL AND INSULIN

What is the role of cortisol and insulin in the metabolism

As mentioned above, cortisol is produced by cholesterol in the two adrenal glands located in the upper part of each kidney. It is usually released in response to events and circumstances such as waking up in the morning, exercising, and acute stress. The long-term systemic effect of cortisol plays an essential role in the body's efforts to perform its processes and maintain homeostasis.

Cortisol also plays an important role in human nutrition. It regulates energy by choosing the right type and quantity of substrate (carbohydrates, fats, or proteins) that the body needs to meet the physiological requirements that are imposed on it. Chronically elevated cortisol levels can have a detrimental effect on weight, immune function, and chronic disease risk.

Cortisol (along with adrenaline) is best known for participating in a fight or flight response and for a temporary increase in energy production at the expense of processes that are not necessary for immediate survival. Consequent hormonal and biochemical imbalances (preferably) are supported by a series of negative feedback-driven by hormones.

The following is a typical example of how the stress response works as a common survival mechanism:

1. A person faces stress.

2. A complex hormonal cascade is formed, and the adrenal glands secrete cortisol.

3. Cortisol prepares the body to react in battle or on the run, flooding it with glucose, providing a direct source of energy for the large muscles.

4. Cortisol inhibits insulin production by trying to prevent glucose storage and by promoting its immediate use.

5. Cortisol constricts the arteries, while adrenaline increases the heart rate, forcing the blood to pump faster and faster.

6. Individual addresses and solution to the situation.

7. Hormone levels return to normal.

EFFECTS ON HIGH CORTISOL LEVELS

The imbalance of blood sugar and diabetes

In difficult conditions, cortisol provides glucose in the body, using protein reserves through liver gluconeogenesis. This energy can help a person fight or escape from a stressful factor. However, long-term high cortisol levels consistently produce glucose, which increases blood sugar levels. This mechanism can theoretically increase the risk of type 2 diabetes, although the causative agent is unknown.

Since cortisol's primary function is to prevent the action of insulin, essentially causing insulin resistance, the body remains completely in insulin resistance when the cortisol level is chronically high. Over time, the pancreas attempts to keep up with the high demand for insulin, blood glucose levels remain high, cells cannot get the sugar they need, and the cycle continues.

Intermittent fasting techniques are most commonly used to help the general population lose weight. The method has been tested by thousands of people and has been scientifically proven to be a useful source of reducing fat and improving body composition.

Weight loss is often considered the most important reason people choose a diet and a program that uses intermittent fasting.

While body fat reduction is one of the best benefits mentioned for intermittent fasting, people get more advantages when choosing this type of program, especially if they work hard to do it and introduce self-control, which will ensure that they do not succumb to thirst. It is well known that intermittent fasting also improves the composition of the body, as previously mentioned.

The body composition refers to a series of characteristics: this applies mainly to fat percentage lean and mass muscle lean. A program that uses intermittent fasting, together with an adequate diet, will reduce the rate of body fat and, at the same time, increase lean muscle mass.

It is also important to consider the benefits of weight loss in people with excessive proliferation of fat in the body since overweight and obesity are associated with so many chronic diseases that can really make your life terrible, and losing even a small weight can drastically reduce the risk of these diseases. Additionally, if you have been diagnosed with an obesity-related illness, weight loss can ease symptoms and help you control your condition.

Take, for example, type 2 diabetes. In one study, scientists describe factors such as pro-inflammatory markers, cytokines, hormones, and esterified increases in glycerol and fatty acids in obese people. In turn, all of these factors have factors that link them to insulin resistance. When insulin resistance develops, it is possible to continue developing type 2 diabetes if they do not take the necessary precautions. When you develop type 2 diabetes, you have a predisposition for many other risks and complications. Type 2 diabetes can cause serious complications, which can lead to disability and be life-threatening. This disease can also affect all major organs in the body, including the heart, and can damage various tissues, such as nerves, throughout the body. In addition to losing weight and reducing the risk of obesity, intermittent fasting has many other benefits worth mentioning.

Through intermittent fasting, cellular changes in the body can occur. This can lead to an increase in growth hormone levels of up to 500%. This leads to faster fat burning and, at the same time, causes an increase in muscle mass.

Intermittent fasting has also been found to help eliminate impurities accumulated in the cells of the human body and can also help repair damaged cells. This means that the body's cells become more efficient in performing their specialized functions.

The study also explains how recent researchers' findings suggest that intermittent fasting helps improve brain health and may play a key role in helping doctors better understand how some diseases such as Parkinson's and Alzheimer's disease can be prevented in the future. Adhering to a fasting plan with breaks can reduce inflammation in the human body and fight oxidative stress. These two factors have a significant impact on many chronic diseases and can cause damage to specific molecules that can inhibit their functioning in the body. In one study, the researchers looked at how intermittent fasting can work in the brain and cardiovascular health in a group of laboratory mice. They found significant improvements in several tests to determine these two most essential body hormones' health status. The researchers also linked these improvements among the laboratory rats tested with the observed reduction in oxidative stress. Also, the researchers observed an improvement in stress resistance levels in these rats. This means that an intermittent fasting diet can help reduce the effects of stress on the body and help fight existing oxidative damage, often also called free radical damage, which has already taken place.

CHAPTER 2 - INTERMITTENT FASTING APPROACH

Lose weight and burn fat.

In most weight-loss diets, they consist of many rules. Fortunately, one of the most popular methods of losing weight on an empty stomach doesn't have many rules or conditions. Intermittent fasting is simple: it is a diet in which one or more meals are tactically skipped over some time. Intermittent fasting does not consist in reducing the calories in a meal, but in skipping the whole meal. That's why it is considered to be one of the simplest diet models. The reasons for the growing popularity of intermittent fasting are:

- A simple dietary pattern

- The effectiveness of the loss of fat belly and loss of weight

- Other health benefits

Intermittent Fasting and Weight Loss

Intermittent fasting, as suggested from the name, it is the diet to fast for a limited period during the day. Fasting usually lasts from 16 to 20 hours, and food is consumed for the remaining 4-8 hours during the day. The fasting period is called the fasting window.

During fasting, you can drink liquids (water, black coffee, herbal teas, etc.). You can see better results if more time is spent per day on an empty stomach. There is no specific image: you can fast as many times as you want. _The faster you are, the more effective the result_. By adhering to fasting, you get additional health benefits in addition to weight loss.

How does your body lose weight during fasting? Your body uses the accumulated body fat (nutritional reserve) for energy and burns all unwanted calories. When you burn calories in this way, you lose weight and burn excess fat. This will help you get a slim figure, and you will also feel healthy and energetic because your body uses excess fat for energy. This is because energy is not obtained from food because consumption is limited. Intermittent fasting helps the body to optimize the release of the main hormones to burn fat, in particular insulin and HGH (human growth hormone), the two most important.

The human growth hormone is responsible for the integration of the body's fat-burning system. Your body starts burning all excess fat to give you energy for further regular (routine) work. Studies show that fasting increases growth hormone (HGH) production by 2000 percent in men and 1,300 percent in women. Intermittent fasting also has a big impact on another important hormone: insulin. It helps maintain a constant and low level of insulin, which is the key to losing excess weight or preventing the accumulation of extra fat in the body. Products rich in processed carbohydrates accumulate in the adipose tissue. Therefore, it is advisable to avoid these foods because it causes a rapid increase in insulin levels and therefore blocks them from each food. This will cause the accumulation of excess fat in the body instead of burning it as energy. When insulin levels rise, they end up with health problems such as obesity, type II diabetes, and other chronic conditions.

Intermittent fasting is the solution to all these problems. Clinical studies have shown that 15 days of continuous, intermittent fasting helps balance insulin levels. Your body remains in a state of fat burning, which gives you more energy during the day.

Nobody wants to lose muscle mass or water content in the body, and most weight-loss diets do this. But studies[1] have shown that fasting helps the body lose more fat and less water or muscle mass. In contrast, most other weight loss regimens do the opposite. The study[2] showed that intermittent fasting helped people cut their waist by 4 to 7 percent in 24 weeks, i.e., the loss of belly fat, the most difficult to burn in the body. Other studies have shown that fasting on alternate days reduced, on average, about 3.8 kg of body fat.

---

[1] https://pubmed.ncbi.nlm.nih.gov/29086496/
[2] https://pubmed.ncbi.nlm.nih.gov/26374764/

Intermittent fasting helps maintain muscle mass.

The main problem associated with most weight loss projects is the loss of fat and muscle, and if you want to experience healthy weight loss, it is essential to maintain your body's muscle mass. It is because muscle maintenance is essential to ensure that the body's metabolic rate does not fall too low. If you don't support your muscles and focus only on fat loss, you can recover lost fat after completing your diet. However, a good protein diet and strength training are the two most important aspects of building muscle mass.

Studies show that around 50 percent of weight gain occurs between November and January during the year. Therefore, if you still control your weight during the holiday season, you don't have to worry about gaining weight. Unfortunately, this isn't easy because it can seem silly when counting calories and macronutrients during a party. But there is a better way! For example, you can skip breakfast and prepare a great Christmas dinner, then prepare a light dinner. The key is to skip a meal or two on the day you plan to celebrate. This way, you don't have to worry about losing your favorite food.

Intermittent fasting doesn't make you feel hungry

The yo-yo effect, also called the cycle of strength, is a repeated increase and decrease in body weight over time. When you introduce your body to a restrictive diet, it causes a change in hunger hormones. For this reason, you can end up with an uncontrollable appetite for food and the severe pain of hunger. Intermittent fasting does not cause the yo-yo effect because the fasting and feeding

18

pattern is divided into intervals. This means that this fasting method can reduce body calories without causing hunger. Intermittent fasting can be a change for you if:

- you want to lose abdominal fat

- you can skip meals without making a fuss

- you want to spend less time cooking and cleaning (lighter notes!)

How effective is intermittent fasting to lose fat?

Intermittent fasting encourages the body to burn more fat. Blood sugar increases at the end of a meal. The blood sugar and glycogen (stored carbohydrates) in your body are energy (your body burns), which is responsible for keeping it alive and functioning healthily. When this happens, your body has no choice but to start burning stored fat for energy.

As told above, body fat is nothing more than accumulating excess calories that accumulate in your body every time you eat too much. The body absorbs all these excess calories and stores them as body fat (nutritional reserve) to be used as a reserve energy source when:

-	It becomes a calorie deficit due to intense exercise or when you eat less.

-	Your body is forced to burn excess calories that accumulate as fat because you don't have enough carbohydrates or blood sugar to burn on an empty stomach for more than 14 hours.

So when your body burns energy, you naturally lose weight because you burn all excess calories. By combining a periodic fast with an appropriate training plan, you lose more fat and weight, which guarantees a slim figure.

The metabolic rate increases when intermittent fasting is observed. This is because when your energy level drops with your blood sugar level, your body reacts oppositely, releasing more adrenaline (norepinephrine). This gives you more energy and allows you to focus on routine work. Since your body releases adrenaline, it forces you to burn all the accumulated fat to provide energy. These stored fats are mainly found in the hips, stomach, and thighs. Indeed, periodic fasting usually affects the area of abdominal fat. It is very difficult to lose abdominal fat because the abdomen area has more alpha-2 receptors (reduces the rate of fat burning) than beta-2 receptors (accelerating fat burning). When intermittent fasting is observed, insulin levels decrease, which closes the A2 receptors (because they cannot function well without insulin) and activates B2 receptors in the abdominal area, allowing the body to burn excess belly fat. The increased blood flow around the abdomen makes fat-burning hormones do a good job. It is possible to reduce the last portion of fat accumulated by the body through intermittent fasting. This fasting method is more important for women because they have more fat (or A2 receptors) on the thighs, buttocks, and hips. As mentioned earlier, growth hormone naturally increases due to intermittent fasting and helps burn more fat.

Here are six popular ways to do it.

1. 16/8 METHOD

This method is the most popular. This means that there is no food for 16 hours a day on an empty stomach, followed by an 8 hour period during which 2-3 meals can be eaten. During fasting, you can drink water or non-caloric drinks such as tea or coffee. Just don't eat anything after dinner, and it will probably take around 16 hours for lunch to arrive the next day. If you are a person who naturally skips breakfast, you can easily apply this method, also known as the "Leangains protocol." Many health experts recommend that women change their diet slightly and eat after 14-15 hours because they improve with a marginally shorter fast. Therefore, it is an effective method to lose weight; it is vital to eat healthy food for 8 hours. The advantages of this method are, among other things: saving money, because you are eating less food; you don't have to count calories and burn fat. One of the difficulties with this method is that it is very strict about what you can and cannot eat. It is suitable for people who consider themselves addicted to gyms, as well as for endurance athletes.

2. EAT-STOP-EAT

To achieve this, do a 24-hour fast once or twice a week. The best way to do this is to skip a meal at the same time the next day. An example would be the end of dinner at 7 pm. The day after, you don't eat before seven. You can also go from breakfast to breakfast or from lunch to lunch if it is more comfortable for your lifestyle. Again, water and other calorie-free drinks are fine. Eat normally while feeding, but look for healthy food. This method requires a lot of self-discipline, but it can be better if you want to normally eat for most of the week and focus on fasting for only one or two days. The benefits of this method include that it requires less willpower. You can also eat anything you want in moderation.

3. METHOD 5: 2

This method is very similar to Eat-Stop-Eat but does not require fasting for 24 hours. To do this, you usually eat five days a week and limit yourself to 500-600 calories a day, twice a week. Some studies suggest that women should consume 500 calories and men up to 600. This is usually divided into two small meals a day. Two days of low-calorie fasting should not be consecutive. Smaller research was conducted with this method, and critics quickly noticed that no scientific studies are confirming its effectiveness, so I can't recommend it. Also, this method requires tracking the calories you eat, so this is a disadvantage.

4. WARRIOR METHOD

You fast all day and then eat at night. It reminds of Vikings movies, in which the warriors return to the cabin and wait for the boxes and dishes with abundant food. During the day, you can eat fruits and vegetables when they are raw. So eat a giant meal at night. Technically, you have a 4-hour window for food at night, but most users of this method hold too much food. This fasting/diet method is compatible with the "Paleo " diet, where people try to keep healthy and natural while eating unprocessed food products similar to those found in nature. Of all the diets that have become popular in recent years, the warriors' diet was the first to contain intermittent fasting. This method's advantages are: 1) You can eat the right snacks and 2) It is very, very healthy. The downside is that you need to control yourself and make sure you choose healthy foods. In addition to raw fruits and vegetables, fast for 20 hours a day. There are some similarities with Ramadan or a 30-day Muslim fast.

5. ALTERNATIVE FASTING DAY

If you are ready for the challenge, you can try fasting every two days. This is a revolutionary method that beginners should not try, but you can opt for a fast or limit your calorie intake to around 500 every two days. This type of method's advantages are 1) rapid weight loss 2) requires less willpower because you eat a little on fasting days and can expect more the next day. The disadvantage is that you have to be very careful not to overeat.

6. SKIPPING MEALS

It is not necessary to follow an extremely rigorous program to obtain the benefits of intermittent fasting. Today's market forces have convinced most of us that we have to eat every few hours. Otherwise, we will lose muscle tension and starve. If you are not hungry or too busy to stop and eat, simply skip the meal. It has only advantages. In general, the human body is previously configured to cope with hunger, so skipping one or two meals will not cause any harm.

Regardless of the chosen intermittent fasting method, it is essential to repeat the following: remember to make the right decisions when choosing food.

MYTHS

Myth # 1: Fasting is the same as hunger

When many people think of fasting, they think of hunger. After all, if you don't eat, you must be hungry. However, this myth is not real. We fast every day for about eight hours while we sleep, but we don't starve. You can also skip the meal in addition to sleep and not starve. In addition to the basic daily fast that we all do, hunger changes our bodies differently from periodic fasting. In the United States, hunger is rare, although there is more uncertainty about food. If you are hungry, you will not eat or eat low-calorie meals for a while. Indeed, the reaction to hunger begins after three days of malnutrition of a sufficient amount of calories (Berg, Tymoczko, and Strye, 2002). During this time, you will lose weight, but you will also damage your body. In this case, your body and your brain know that you are starving and decide to save you. Your brain slows down your metabolism and sends hormones, so you are very hungry. Your body is starting to look for food elsewhere. Now the science of hunger is very detailed, but suffice it to say that our body usually draws energy from our food, which increases the blood sugar and insulin that feed our body. However, when we starve, our body has no glucose reserves and starts looking for other sources of energy. In search of protein, your body cannibalizes by eating important cells and muscles. This is not a quick process because your body still needs to function to find more food. However, without food, your body slowly loses its functionality, which leads to death. Most of us will not starve in the United States. Even if we use a low-calorie diet, our body will continue to put pressure on us to eat and have high access to food. Even though most of them are unhealthy, they probably don't starve. However, we still feel the effects of hunger reactions without proper nutrition during the day. Our brains will not only continue to send warnings about hunger but will also change emotions and sometimes cognition. Researchers during World War II studied hunger to determine how our bodies respond. This study is known as the Minnesota famine experiment (Keys et al., 1950). They discovered some interesting effects of the famine. Many participants experienced emotional and cognitive changes and dreamed of eating. They physically felt fluctuations in body temperature, felt weak and had reduced resistance. Their heart rates were also decreased. These effects were felt during the hunger phase in which they ate, but only a little every day and very little of what they ate was healthy. Intermittent fasting is something completely different from hunger because you won't spend three days without food. As long as you follow a pre-established, healthy, and fasting program, you will be left without food for only 24 hours or less. So why not start with your natural hunger response. Our body is used to normal fasting, to the states of food. When you eat your last meal before fasting, your body has high blood sugar levels and an increase in insulin that feeds your body.

The body also stores extra glucose and reserves it for later. After the first few hours, your body starts lowering your insulin and blood sugar levels. His liver releases its glucose deposits, and then the body starts using fat to continue feeding, and its blood sugar level is lower. This condition is known as ketosis. Your body remains in this state for a while, even when you eat again (Berg, Tymoczko, and Strye, 2002). Since you supply food to your body, even after 24 hours without it, your body does not change its response to hunger. Instead, it adheres to the stage of ketosis, with levels of reduced insulin and blood sugar, before you get more energy from the next meal.

Remember that although there are differences between hunger and fasting, any attitude that is too long will cause hunger. Any diet that consumes less than 1,000 calories per day exposes you to hunger reactions. As long as you eat something during the day, you will be fine. In most meals, you consume your usual calories daily. But in some meals, such as 5: 2 fasting and on alternate days, you will have periods of reduced calorie intake. Even in these periods, you will be without food for 24 hours or less. During intermittent fasting, your body should not respond to hunger.

Myth # 2: fasting makes you increase weight

This myth is closely related to the previous myth. This is related to the response to hunger or the number of people who call it "hunger modality.".

We've already discussed how fasting won't put you in hunger mode if you do it correctly. Let's explore the aspect of metabolism after hunger, and the body/mind will start to save energy by first reducing the metabolism. Your metabolism helps maintain body weight and repair cells. In this way, your body processes the food you eat and transforms it into fuel used to speed up all your activities. During hunger, the metabolic rate decreases because you don't have enough food to keep it optimal. This is to save energy on the most important vital functions. People often think that fasting is hunger. They expect their metabolism to slow down during fasting, which increases their weight. This is confusing because during hunger, yes, the metabolic rate decreases, but your body uses all the reserves it has. This means there is no additional fuel! You will not gain weight when you starve. It's impossible to transfer this belief to this method. You will hear people talk about "fast" and "slow" metabolism in most food cultures. Fast metabolism should help you lose weight because you burn more food and fuel than you eat and store. Slow metabolism is assumed to cause weight gain because too little fuel is consumed, and everything you eat is stored. When people think about this myth, they think that their lack of food will reduce their metabolism, which will lead to greater food storage, lower energy consumption, and savings. Fasting improves metabolism and effectively uses energy resources (Patterson et al., 2016). You will likely lose weight during fasting and not gain weight. Although I would like to discredit this myth completely, there is some truth in it, and it all comes down to diet.

You can gain weight during fasting, but this is not due to your metabolic rate. If you decide to eat regular meals that exceed daily calories, you will gain weight. It is the same with every diet, fasting, and food. If you exceed the amount consumed by your body in terms of energy/food, you will gain weight. But if so, it is not due to a lower metabolic rate, but more because of a poorly planned diet, and to avoid this, it is important to eat balanced nutritious meals. This will help you maintain weight or lose something, even if it is a change in your normal diet. You can also combine calorie restriction with your meal, and we will discuss it in the next chapter. If you gain weight during fasting, you should monitor what you eat.

Myth # 3: fasting is not sustainable in the long term

There are so many unbalanced diets. I'm thinking now of a diet in which only one type of food is consumed; for example, a diet based on cabbage. These types of diets are not balanced because it is easy to start eating multiple types of food. Your body will crave the nutrients it needs until you are bored with this type of food. Many trendy diets are unbalanced because they often do not provide the body with the requirements for proper functioning. This makes you hungry and thirsty for forbidden foods in these diets. Fasting is not like fashion, and it does not limit certain types of food. So even if you are hungry, you prefer not to have brutal desires.

Also, there are many types of fasting. Some of these are easy to integrate into everyday life, such as the 14/10 or 16/8 protocol. Thanks to these diets, you simply prolong your fasting beyond the normal eight hours of sleep. Sometimes this means eating the last early meal or the first late meal. Since these two types are simple and easy to implement, they can also be easy to maintain.

Myth # 4: fasting causes are overeating

This myth is based somehow on reality. This is due to how often we react when we skip a meal. We all know this feeling. You decided to work for lunch and starve before going home. You approach the pantry and start eating everything that fills the void and ends hunger. When we arrive, we are surrounded by the remains of what we have eaten. It can be very surprised how much you have eaten for some time, which seems like a desperate hunger.

What can be doubly surprising is that during this almost insatiable feeling of hunger, our bodies send signals that tell us to eat, but after a while, they also stop. Unfortunately, many of us hear the "I'm full" signal from our brain when we are in this state. So we eat too much. This is certainly a typical binge feeling. If we get to the point where we are very hungry, we often start eating everything we have, and it is very difficult for us to stop. So yes, you can bite when you stop chatting during your first meal. But this doesn't have to happen, and it doesn't happen to many people. This is because people understand how hunger works and how to stop fasting properly to avoid overeating. When you break the fast, you want to relax. Depending on the type of meal, it can be stored after 14 hours or 24 hours. That's why it's important to stop fasting. Don't clog up with everything you see. Take a deep breath. Drink coffee or tea. So start eating with something small. Take a short break and then eat a little more. Listen to the "I'm full" sign of your body. So stop eating. One way that can help this feeling is to be more careful when eating.

Mindfulness is a common term today, but it can be used for food.

With the utmost attention, you can determine what total feeling means for your body. You can find out when to slow down and stop eating. Remember to eat to pay attention to the signs of hunger. All of these things can help you break your fast without fear. There is some truth in this myth, but it is easy to manage and prevent.

CHAPTER 3 – THE 16/8 METHOD STEP BY STEP

Now is the time to get into the real nitty-gritty that this method is based on. We have said that there are many different intermittent protocols, and some ask you to fast for 24 hours.

The 16: 8 methods differ from others because there are no long and tedious fasts; you fast only for 16 hours a day and normally eat for 8 hours. Now it sounds a lot, 16 hours, but you will sleep more on time! See, you can move the fasting period according to your needs. We'll talk about how to proceed in more detail soon, but a good example is someone who needs breakfast compared to someone who doesn't want to eat early in the morning. We are all different, but most of us fall into one of these two categories. You can wake up to breakfast hungry and in need; otherwise, you cannot concentrate. Alternatively, you can wake up enough to make a coffee and feel a bit 'sick' if you eat right away. If necessary, you can have breakfast as soon as you wake up, starting from the period of its 8-hour power.

If you don't want to eat after waking up, you can get up, get dressed, drink sugar-free black coffee, and skip breakfast, starting at lunch. For example, you will begin eating at 12:00. This means that you can eat freely until 20:00. So you can sleep at 22:00.

The 16: 8 methods are so popular. Of course, during the 8-hour feeding period, you should consider what you eat. If you fill these 8 hours with chips and chocolate, you will eat a lot more calories than you should for 24 hours a day, and you will probably gain weight instead of losing! However, if you are aware of what you eat without being particularly restrictive, but only think about the health line, you will be full and satisfied at the end of the window with the food. This means that you will lose weight fairly easily and also get the general benefits of intermittent fasting. See how easy it can be?

HOW TO USE INTERMITTENT FASTING TO LOSE WEIGHT

You learned about the benefits of 16: 8 intermittent fasting, and now you can ask how exactly this type of weight loss fasting program is used. I have good and bad news here. The process of using intermittent fasting to get rid of excess fat is quite simple, but only if you have the right tools and tips. You can't just start fasting and keep eating as many doughnuts as you can when you get to the window to eat. This is a recipe for disaster. You end up gaining weight instead of losing weight! In this part, I will tell you more about using intermittent fasting, along with the appropriate diet and program, to make sure you can burn calories to lose weight. I will divide the whole process into several stages to better understand where to start and how it should work to achieve the desired results.

How is weight loss generally achieved? Before examining the best way to use intermittent fasting to reduce body fat percentage, let's first think about how weight loss in general works and consider it an effective and guaranteed scientific weight-loss method. When you eat something, whatever it is, the calories are put into your body. Your body breaks down and absorbs nutrients when carbohydrates are broken down and then converted into glucose, which is then distributed throughout the body to provide energy to the cells. When excess glucose is present in your body, it is usually stored as fat cells in a rather complicated process, which we will not discuss in detail here. When fat cells increase, you gain weight, which ultimately leads to overweight and therefore slows down obesity.

On the other hand, when you are physically active, you burn calories by walking, dancing, or putting a lot of effort into the gym tape. Your body uses more glucose to produce energy, and when the reserves run out, the body starts looking at the stored fat cells to generate more energy. This energy allows you to continue running on this stick or lift a set of weights several times. To sum up: eat, collect calories; if you train, you lose calories. When the amount of calories consumed exceeds the number of calories lost, you will gain weight. Think about it within 24 hours. If you eat 2,000 calories but only consume 1,000, you will gain weight up to 1,000 more calories at the end of the day. When you eat more calories than you burn, it means excess calories. Thanks to this strategy, you gain weight, and you cannot lose weight. To lose weight, the whole equation must be reversed. You have to lose more calories than you burn. If you eat products that calculate around 2,000 calories per day, you must burn over 2,000 calories if you want the fat to disappear, and the number of scales decreases. When your daily calorie intake is less than the number of calories you lose, you have a calorie deficit: this is the ideal goal for which you strive to reduce weight.

HOW TO APPLY THE 16: 8 METHODS QUICKLY

• Eat for 8 hours a day, one at a time: you can't divide these hours, look at them as a block of time

• Quickly for 16 hours a day, once again, do it in sequence

• You can choose when to take your eight-block food hours, but a good idea to continue at the same times every day so that the body can get used or adjust to the routine.

• All the times after must coincide with sleep to reduce the number of conscious messages.

• Do not be afraid to miss breakfast as this routine does not have an "important" food "day, but only one important window to eat.

• You can drink tea, coffee, and black coffee without sugar, water, and other drinks that do not contain calories freely during the day. It is time to eat and fast, and you should consume enough water during the day to prevent dehydration.

• During feeding, you should carefully divide your meals to avoid catching up when you stop fasting initially. It will only cause stomach pain and other unpleasant stomach symptoms!

• Choose healthy meals as much as possible, but there is no limit to what you can eat. However, if you are not healthy, remember that you will not create the calorie deficit needed for weight loss.

• Although you don't need to count calories when using the 16: 8 method, you can consider standard calories, which is an average of 2,500 for a man and an average of 2,000 for a woman.

• You should also exercise if you want to get additional health benefits and accelerate weight loss.

• Never try to reduce the feeding window or reduce calories below average; It will lead to extreme hunger. Remember that fasting is not starving!

WHAT YOU CAN AND CANNOT EAT

Again, there are no rules on what you can eat and what you cannot eat; this is a completely free option, following a 16: 8 diet. However, you should consider your overall health in the options you should consider healthy compared to unhealthy; the idea is to create a calorie deficit during the entire 24 hour period. To do this, remember to fast and eat in the right proportion of time, for example, 8 hours of food and 16 hours of fasting, and follow the healthy options available during meals. Thanks to this, you will feel infinitely better. If you want to know something about the healthiest products that you can even include in your day, take a look at the list below.

• Eggs: remember to eat egg yolk because it contains vitamins and proteins!

• Green leaves: we are talking about things like spinach, chard, cabbage, and Swiss, to name a few, and these are rich in fiber and also have few calories

• Fatt fish like salmon - Salmon is a fish that will keep you filled, but is also rich in omega-three fatty acids, which are excellent for improving brain health, reducing inflammation, and general, also help you lose weight. If you don't like salmon, try mackerel, trout, herring, and sardines.

• Cruciferous vegetables: in this case, look at Brussels sprouts, broccoli, cabbage, and cauliflower. Again, these types of vegetables contain a large amount of fiber, which helps you feel longer, but they also have the properties to fight cancer.

• Lean meat: stick to beef and chicken for the best options, but remember to choose thinner cuts. Possible here, you will get a good protein enhancer, but you can also prepare all kinds of delicious dishes from both types of meat!

• Boiled potatoes: you may think that potatoes are harmful to you, and in most cases, they are, especially if you fry them, but boiled potatoes are a good option, especially if there is a shortage of potassium. They are also very full.

• Tuna: this type of fish differs from the bluefish listed above and is very low in fat but rich in protein. Choose a healthier canned tuna that contains water instead of oil. Put it on a potato jacket for a tasty and healthy meal!

• Beans and other types of legumes: they form the basis of any healthy diet and are also very abundant. We are talking about beans, lentils, and black beans, which are rich in fiber and protein.

• Ricotta: if you are a fan of cheese, there is no reason to deny it, but most cheeses have enough fat. If so, why not choose ricotta? It is high in protein and abundant, but low in calories.

• Avocado: today's trendy food is very healthy and excellent for increasing brainpower! Add a toast to a wonderful breakfast rich in potassium and lots of fiber.

• Walnuts: instead of eating chocolate and chips, why not eat walnuts? You will receive large quantities of healthy fats, fiber, and proteins, as well as filling. However, don't overeat because they can be high in calories if exceeded.

I try to turn it on and off quickly. For starters, try quinoa, brown rice, and oatmeal.

• Fruit: not all fruits are healthy, but they are certainly a better option than chocolate and fries! You will also receive many different vitamins and minerals and an injection of antioxidants in your diet, which is perfect for your immune system.

• Seeds: Again, like nuts, seeds are an excellent snack and can be sprinkled with many dishes, such as yogurt and porridge. Try chia seeds for low-calorie, high-fiber treatments.

• Coconut oil and extra virgin olive oil: you've certainly heard of the wonders of coconut oil, and this is very healthy cooking oil. Coconut oil is produced from so-called medium-chain triglycerides, and although I can panic from the word triglycerides, they are a healthy type! However, if you want to buy something completely healthy, you cannot beat virgin olive oil.

• Whole grains: everyone knows that whole grains are full of fiber and therefore keep them longer, so it is the perfect option for anyone who wants to stop quickly. For starters, try quinoa, brown rice, and oatmeal.

• Yogurt: ideal for improving intestinal health, yogurt is your friend because it will provide you with a complete level and contain the content of probiotics, as long as you are looking for products with the words "live and active cultures "on your plate.

Avoid too sweet yogurt snacks, and anything that says "low fat" isn't as positive as it sounds! There are many delicious dishes to try, and you can easily create tasty recipes from one of these ingredients! A little later in the book, we will show you some recipes to see how easy healthy eating is and how satisfying it can be.

So what should you not eat? There is nothing beyond borders, but the point is how much you eat. If you want a slice of pizza, you can eat it, but make sure you only have a healthier diet for the rest of the day. Remember that one of the reasons why fasting is so popular is because you don't move your finger when you occasionally grab a chocolate bar. You don't have to feel guilty because you're hungry for hamburgers once a week, as long as you know that moderation has to be inside.

What exactly is moderation? You know when to stop, and you know what enough is and what's too much. For example, enjoying a pizza in moderation not mean several pieces of pizza once a week. You can still enjoy what you like, but you don't always have it.

Here is an example of a diet for this fasting method:

The first day it's time to wake up: you can drink coffee, tea (without calories, without sugar) or water, whatever you choose

Stick to liquids like water, coffee, and tea and natural calorie-free sweeteners like Stevia and Xylitol. Lunch: chicken breast with many green leafy vegetables or another protein source, such as meat, pork, fish, or turkey. Try adding good fats like coconut or avocado. Snacks: nuts and seeds are excellent snacks during the day. Dinner: salmon (or another healthy source of fish or protein) with vegetables. Before bedtime: try to stop eating two hours before bedtime.

Day 2 Wake up: just like the first day, coffee or tea (no calories) so you can move when needed. Keep the same liquids as day 1. Select natural, non-artificial sweeteners again. Lunch: vegetable protein. Snacks: nuts, seeds, or berries. Lunch the same two-hour window for one or two small meals. Try the roasted chicken breast with roasted vegetables. Before bedtime: I always try to wait two hours after eating to go to sleep.

Your diet will mainly contain unprocessed foods. Meat, fish, eggs, vegetables, and only a small amount of fruit with a low glycemic index should mainly consist of meals. Processed foods are generally rich in heat and have a low nutritional value.

Drink lots of water. Try to take at least 1/2 ounce per day for every pound of body weight. (For example, 130 pounds per person would use around 2 liters per day and about 3 liters per person who weighs 190 pounds.) It looks like a lot of water, but it's useful for keeping your skin full and hydrated. The average person generally thinks he is hungry when he is thirsty. Drinking water will help stop hunger. You can also chew sugarless gum to give your lips something to do. Studies have shown that some gums have some sweeteners that turn into calories in the stomach, so you should stick to the sugar-free variety. Traditionally, most instructors and trainers recommend a hearty breakfast or 4-5 balanced meals throughout the day. The 16/8 method skips breakfast as an extension of natural fasting for the night. Sitting and hunger will make it more difficult for you to move. The 16/8 method is often used in combination with a rigorous training regimen and, as such, should be used in combination with a branched-chain amino acid. If you combine a 16/8 intermittent fast with an intense training regimen, you may want to add more protein for dinner. So search for protein animal or vegetable protein supplements.

Possible defect related to intermittent fasting

Every diet has advantages and disadvantages. The most significant disadvantage of intermittent fasting is that you have to fast for a few days for it to work! The advantage of the 16:8 method, as you will find, is that you can stretch them easily to make sure you sleep most of the time, so it's much less noticeable. You can also transfer the meal period to your preferred time. It doesn't matter when you fast, as long as you follow the rules and fast for the right time below. Of course, fasting at first will make you hungry. This cannot be avoided.

It can be annoying at first, but you will find ways to deal with them, such as distraction techniques, late gratification, and drinking water. In most cases, when we think we are hungry, we are not really; usually, we are bored and even thirsty. During fasting, you can drink water and even drink sugar-free black tea or coffee, which can relieve hunger.

The biggest challenge that many people face when starting a periodic fast is not overeating while eating. When you have fasted x the number of hours, you will be hungry when you start eating. This may mean that you are open to the bigger meal, regardless of its content. Remember that intermittent fasting doesn't tell you what you can and can't eat, but you still have to eat healthily. There is no diet on this planet that allows you to eat french fries, pizza, chocolate, and all the sweet pastries and carbohydrates you usually want because they stimulate you to gain weight again! You can quickly get a strange offer when you fast from time to time, but you will have to avoid developing it to overdo it when the fast ends.

You will probably soon realize that if there is excess after fasting, the stomach will say it out loud and perhaps spectacularly in a way that you don't accept! A too heavy meal after fasting can cause stomach pain, gas, and discomfort. It is best to store light foods and accumulate them over time. Developing willpower and knowing the difference between healthy eating and terrible eating will be something you will learn quickly enough. Still, the fact is that the restriction can often mean that people with less self-discipline can fall into the trap larger. There is also a fear that women will find it more difficult than men. All of this is due to hormones. Women are much more sensitive to calorie fluctuations than men because they have different hormones. This means that when calories are limited, hormone levels change. When hormone levels change, side effects can occur. The good news is that the 16: 8 methods we are talking about are among the best intermittent fasting methods for women because they don't significantly affect hormones. Some other methods, i.e., types that require fasting during the day, or sometimes during the week, often cause hormonal disturbances in women. In most cases, you can control any side effect by choosing the right method

HOW TO AVOID BAD EATING HABITS

I mentioned it briefly, but it's worth repeating; you can't eat junk all the time. Like everything else in life, you will go out quickly, stopping what you impose. If you want to lose weight with fasting breaks, you will be more successful and get faster results by eating healthy food. Discussing all the details on healthy foods' appearance is beyond this book's goal, but we all know what it means — processed foods to eat less and for "whole" food. If you want to avoid the package or box's food, you need to remove processed food. It takes longer to prepare and plan, but if you plan on eating less food, you should make the food you eat important for your body. Intermittent fasting is not a free pass to eat what you want. Avoid this trap when planning. Sometimes it is difficult to plan meals, but it is better not to finish eating a hamburger or cook something in the microwave that looks like food.

Who wouldn't be happy with all the benefits that can come from an interrupted fast? The problem with all this enthusiasm can mean that you jump to the bottom without learning to swim. Your body has adapted to the normal feeding rhythm. When you break it, your body will tell you. Your body will be more aggressive in understanding that you are playing with its rhythm. Hunger pain, headache, dizziness, irritability, weakness, and discomfort are just some of the symptoms that appear when your body tells you that there are no hours if you jump on the bottom. Avoiding all of this is as easy as relaxing from the start, no matter how difficult it is when you get excited. This gives your body time to adjust to the new feeding rhythm and learn to feel normal during fasting, so you know when something is wrong, and you have to check it again.

You only think about food and hunger.

The majority of us have spent a lot of time because we were very hungry before we start fasting. When we begin to discover what true hunger is, it is not always difficult to think about the food and hunger we have. It is a process that everyone goes through. No matter how strong your will is, at first, you will be hungry and think a lot about food. This is normal, and most people go through it without much pain. At first, it can be overwhelming and prevent you from following the chosen method of intermittent fasting. The best way to avoid it is to take care of it. Do the things you like in order to avoid thinking about food. I recommend leaving home because it is always easy to find food when you are at home, and you may already have the habit of eating snacks while watching TV or a hobby. Try to avoid the things you usually do when eating meals.

Fast too long.

The general idea of intermittent fasting is that you do it in small quantities. Although studies are suggesting that occasional fasting is good, it should not be repeated multiple times. "More is better" is not a motto. Intermittent fasting is stressful for your body. These mild stressors are good as long as you have enough time to recover. As with weight lifting, you can't wait for better results if you don't have time to recover. When you put too much stress on your body, you last longer and don't have enough time to recover; you will see diminishing returns and it will start doing more harm than good. If you stop fasting long enough, you will want to cross the boundaries of these plans because you will see the results, and your body will treat it physically and mentally. The solution to this problem is to recognize that the methods described in this book are tried, true, and designed for some reason. No method requires fasting for more than one day at a time. Although each method can be customized to your needs, remember that there are restrictions on the stress your body can endure before it stops being beneficial.

Abuse of coffee.

Many people sometimes rely too much on coffee to fill the break between meals. Coffee is excellent for this, but be careful not to become addicted to coffee. Caffeine is a stimulant, and you can easily become addicted to it if you abuse it to overcome it. If you drink coffee all day because you're too hungry, you've probably done it too early. I don't deny that coffee saves lives, but you shouldn't rely on it to end the fast. Caffeine has a half-life of 6 hours. This means those 6 hours after drinking the coffee, and it still has half the effect of the first drink. Twelve hours after drinking, coffee still has ¼ of its potency. With that in mind, it's easy to understand why you should limit the amount of coffee you drink and how late it is to drink it during the day. This can significantly affect sleep cycles and overall health. Since it's about weight loss and improved health, it's best to control coffee consumption. You can avoid issues by limiting the number of cups a day to one or two and making sure you don't drink coffee in the afternoon. We all have days when we need extra energy to spend, but this shouldn't be the habit of drinking too much coffee or the afternoon.

You don't drink enough water

The body needs extra water during fasting for several reasons. First, it helps you feel fuller by putting something in your stomach. This is also necessary because while your body is not focusing its energy on digesting food during the day; It breaks cells and creates new ones. This accelerated healing process leads to an unusual amount of cellular debris that needs to be removed. Adequate hydration allows the body to make this process as efficient as possible. In addition to removing cellular debris, the body breaks down fat reserves to produce energy during fasting. The toxins that we find every day accumulate in our fat deposits, and when we break down the fat cells, we get a very strong dose of these toxins. It is extremely important to be well hydrated when it happens so that toxins are removed from the body and do not accumulate elsewhere or cause harm. When people get dizzy and have headaches during fasting, they come from blood toxins that need to be eliminated. To avoid this, you should focus on drinking lots of water during fasting. On fasting days, drink at least two liters (or eight glasses) of water per day. Even if you don't drink water, you have to start. If necessary, try drinking water throughout the day. You will appreciate the lack of headaches during fasting.

You are always afraid of hunger

It is worth remembering again because, in the beginning, it is difficult to beat. Accidental hunger is normal and healthy for the body. You can spend weeks without food, drinking enough water. The hunger felt during the hours or on the day of the fast is manageable and will improve over time. If you are working on a more rigorous fasting method, don't let the fear of hunger stop you. It will pass, and you will survive. Intermittent fasting benefits are too great to allow for occasional hunger that prevents you from reaching your goals. You can prevent and control this fear by overwhelming it, starting slowly and gradually increasing the time to fast. Your body will not eat backward during fasting. All you need is practice to develop this random hunger tolerance.

Eat too little before going to bed

Fasting meals will be bigger than usual, and if you finish fasting for dinner, you will eat a big dinner. The problem is that eating a big meal before dinner can disturb sleep. There are several reasons. First, when your body works hard to digest a big meal, it can increase body temperature and make you feel uncomfortable lying under the bed and trying to sleep. Digestion causes an exothermic reaction. This means that the reaction between the acid in the stomach and food causes heat. The more food reacts, the more heat will be released. The increase in body temperature decreases with the elimination of food in the stomach during the digestive process. In addition to being warm before bedtime, if you consume a large number of carbohydrates before bedtime, your body will release a large amount of insulin into the blood. This insulin can reduce the effect of the explosion of growth hormones released in the first half of the sleep cycle. This makes the improving process difficult. Intermittent fasting should improve sleep unless you eat too close to sleep.

You are a social dining room

One of the most difficult things faced by people who intervene quickly is not hunger, but the social situations in which people usually eat. If you plan to have lunch with colleagues regularly and start a fast that includes skipping lunch, it can be difficult. Lunch is not the only thing lost, but also social interaction with colleagues, which is a problem at the beginning. You have to give up on daily dinners and lose the social interaction that most people expect in the middle of the day, or sit back and drink water while everyone else is eating. There are many situations in which most of us find ourselves in the week; we eat socially, and it would be "strange" if we didn't. Whether with family, friends, or colleagues, hunger leads us to eat many meals. You can do many things to solve this situation. You can completely avoid this situation and simply not participate in the social environments in which people will eat. You can justify yourself by telling people you've just eaten or found another reasonable excuse, or you can tell people that you're always close to what you're doing so they understand why you don't eat, but be prepared for anything. Some comments can be made to convince you that you are doing something unhealthy. What you choose will be the best for you. You must learn to defend yourself and do what is best for you, regardless of what people say or hear. You will be surprised at the frequency with which they offer you cookies at work or invite you to something where people will eat when you start fasting. We rarely think about what's going on, and respecting fasting makes us aware of and helps reduce excess calories from food in the community.

You think intermittent fasting is magical

It is easy to see all the benefits of intermittent fasting and to see that it is magical. We are still working on physiology, even if we optimize this process. This is not a magic weight-loss medicine. It still takes time and effort on your part, although less time and effort than many other weight loss methods. You will get results if you stay with intermittent fasting, but it won't happen overnight. Intermittent fasting is an extraordinary way to lose weight and improve your overall health, so be excited. Just remember that this is a process limited by your body and that no magic goes beyond what it can do.

CHAPTER 4 - THE 16/8 METHOD FROM BEGINNER TO EXPERT

This particular method is especially useful for beginners who fast for the first time. It has less risk, and you will spend less time trying to figure out when the best time to eat is and what you should eat exactly. Various intermittent fasting techniques have been developed, some of which are quite complex and require many preliminary plans to avoid malnutrition or other possible complications. In this book, we focus on the 16: 8 methods, as I said earlier. The reason is simple: the 16: 8 method offers a good overview and a sense of what gives you a fast intermittent and a solid work plan. This is the simplest option that you can choose and does not make you feel hungry.

THE 16/8 METHOD FOR BEGINNERS

The 16: 8 methods are the easiest to follow and understand, so many beginners choose it. Of course, this isn't suitable for everyone, and since one size isn't suitable for everyone, some people can switch to another method after a short time. Okay, this could be something you want to think about. Shortly after that, we'll cover some alternative methods, so always remember that if you find that the 16:8 protocol doesn't work the way you want, then there are other alternatives. However, for the most part, the 16:8 method is very effective for many people and is a method that encourages healthy eating without restrictions or rules. There are big changes in the lifestyle that many people struggle with when trying a different diet, such as Keto, Atkins, Paleo diets, etc. They contain many rules and recipes, as well as a list of what you can eat and not eat and how to prepare. This can overwhelm many beginners and make them rebel and say, "No, thanks!" The 16: 8 method and many other intermittent fasting methods have no rules. You don't have to weigh or count. Just make healthy decisions that aren't surprising. For example:

- Pizza is bad; whole wheat bread is better
- Chocolate is bad; the fruit is better.
- The pies are bad, the vegetables are good.

Can you see how easy it is? Making healthy choices isn't rocket science, and that doesn't mean you always have to be 100% healthy!

Do you want a hamburger? Take one, but only once a week, and make sure the rest of the day is full of healthy food.

The second advantage is that the 16: 8 method shouldn't interfere with your social life. Most people sometimes want to go out with friends or a partner for dinner and go out for a drink, but it can be very difficult to follow a low-calorie or trendy diet. With the 16: 8 method, all you have to do is make an appointment in the eating window. It may be more difficult if you start eating early and end early, but you can always meet for lunch instead of dinner! There is no limit to what you can eat, but you can always make healthy choices on the regular menu in most restaurants. If your window finishes eating a little later, then you have a wider time range.

We summarize the main reasons why most beginners choose the 16: 8 method:

• It is easy to follow and requires no counting, weighing or monitoring

• You can change the feeding schedule according to your needs

• You can set up an important part of the fasting period while you sleep, so you don't notice it so often

• The feeding method must not interfere too much with social life.

• You have no limits to what you can eat as long as you make healthy decisions

• It doesn't look like a diet and a new lifestyle with schedules of foods you can or can't eat

• You can still drink calories, water, and tea or black coffee without sugar

• You won't feel so hungry for this type of nutrition plan because it is not a very long post.

It depends on you! We've already discussed the two main methods that most people try at 16:8, namely skipping breakfast and starting food at lunchtime or for someone who needs breakfast because they can't concentrate without it. Not only when you can eat, but also what you eat. Even if there are no restrictions or lists of foods, you should eat and foods you shouldn't, always remember that you will end up with a stomach ache if you suddenly have a big breakfast or lunch on a plate. This may mean that you end up eating too many calories in the feeding window and gaining weight, or you have stomach problems for the rest of the feeding window. During this period, you don't have enough fuel because the stomach is too swollen; you can't bear the food, and therefore you are hungry during fasting. It is a matter of careful choice, which we will discuss later.

How many calories should you eat? It depends on whether you want to lose weight or keep it. The standard calories for weight maintenance are 2500 calories per day for a man and 2000 calories per day for a woman. It depends on the person's height, current weight, and metabolism; in fact, it is only an average and healthy amount. If you need stronger guidelines in certain circumstances, talk to your doctor, who can provide you with a calorie program tailored to your needs. As part of this amount of calories, it is necessary to ensure a good and varied diet. This means proteins, carbohydrates, fats, vitamins, and minerals. Again, we will discuss what you can and cannot eat in general because there are no rules, but the procedure is different. Ironically, it will help you to enjoy your new life more because you're not bored and don't always eat the same food.

Using the 16: 8 method, you should also drink plenty of water during the day, both on an empty stomach and during meals. This ensures that you do not dehydrate, and it also supports digestion. Also, you should train! Now there are no rules you should exercise according to routine posts, but it will help you lose weight faster and enhance your overall health and well-being. Exercise is fantastic on many levels and helps build lean muscle mass, increasing the ability to burn fat as a source of energy. Exercise is also known to help with problems like anxiety, depression, and stress. We all live a stressful life, and sometimes just a little exercise will bring them out of extremely difficult levels. In addition to everything else, exercise can be social and fun!

THE 16/8 METHOD FOR EXPERT

If you are thinking of introducing an intermittent publishing protocol to lose weight, this may be one of the best decisions you will make. There are many advantages and disadvantages to intermittent fasting. It is best to spend some time, analyze and examine carefully before getting involved.

This protocol has three main advantages and three main disadvantages that I have encountered for over two and a half years of fasting and research.

Pro #1. Weight and fat loss are easier to achieve.

Weight loss is probably the number one reason people start getting a quick result. Personally, my main motivation was fat loss. Although my diet and activity level was good, I wanted to lose more body fat.

Pro #2. Save more time.

Planning six healthy meals a day can be quite stressful. Even planning three meals a day can be a hassle.

If you only eat 7 to 14 meals a week, you can simplify your life in one way, and you can't imagine it. When it starts to, I suggest quickly.

Go food shopping on the same day and time every week. This will help you breakfasting with healthy foods.

Pro #3 It promotes a better general message of health and life expectancy.

Research on fasting and longevity is preliminary but promising: Besides, for protection against diseases such as " obesity and diabetes, fasting can reduce the risk of Alzheimer's and Parkinson's diseases.

If you get sick frequently, fasting can strengthen the immune system if you run a healthy lifestyle.

The first weeks are the most difficult. As with all good things, fasting has its drawbacks. After starting quickly, the first few weeks or months will be the most difficult. If you get used to the continuous for the whole day, and then you stop, your body will be taken by panic.

During this transition period, it is important to take it easy. I am switching from eating all day to once a day is probably not the best solution. I suggest:

Start with the 16/8 protocol: as I said before.

Drink lots of water while fasting: water will help with hunger. The addition of the small "salt" also helps the removal of toxins.

Even if you fast for 12 to 14 hours, it's a good start. It is possible to switch to longer fasting periods gradually. Make sure you eat the right amount of calories - It's easy to get the extreme calorie deficit intermittent fasting. Make sure your meals are abundant and nutritious. Other healthy living practices, such as sleeping well and meditating, will help you overcome it.

Know that you are going through a learning curve and that it will adapt over time.

If you suffer from a disordered diet, it is best to heal before fasting. Fasting can worsen the symptoms of an eating disorder.

Over time, you will want less junk food. You will need a nutritious and warm meal.

When you stop IF, I recommend:

- Fill first with fruit and vegetables.
- Eat as slowly as possible. First help, it will be easier.
- Drink water before meals to reduce overeating.
- Drink kombucha to aid digestion.
- Save up to eating carbohydrates in the end.

If you are constantly in excess, it is best to take a few days off and restock.

***

An example of a day of intermittent fasting 16/8

Breakfast:

- Green Tea, Herbal Tea, Coffee, Water, Water with lemon (for those who like it without problems)

Lunch: (to be eaten at 12:00)

- Pasta (preferably wholemeal) + Protein (meat/fish/egg/vegetable protein such as tofu or tempeh or legumes) + Raw or cooked vegetables + 1 tablespoon of extra virgin olive oil + 1 Fruit of the season (for those who do not have problems with abdominal bloating).

Snack:

- Fresh fruit in season + 10gr dried fruit + rusks or spelled biscuits (n°2)

Dinner: (to be eaten before 20:00)

- Fish or Meat (preferably white) or eggs or vegetable protein + Whole wheat bread (50-70gr) + 1 tablespoon of extra virgin olive oil. (possibly 20gr of 70% dark chocolate).

N.B. Hydrate very well during the day.

Solve problems

As with any goal, especially for improving health, you probably have problems. After hitting an obstacle, it is easy to throw a towel and give up. But please don't do this. When it comes to joining a specific meal calendar, it can be difficult, but the reward is well worth it. So even if you fight, try to continue. In this part, we will discuss some areas where you may have difficulties and ways to recover to continue.

If you find fasting difficult, there may be several problems. Maybe you're not following a good schedule or jumping too fast without giving your body time to adapt. Both can hinder the perfection of fasting. To fix this, go back to the registry and check what you've done so far. So change some things. You can pause the voice and start again by slowly entering the voice. You can also try changing the food and the windows fast. It can also reduce fasting times and stay within 12 hours of fasting and 12 hours of food for several months. You can increase up to 14 hours of fasting and 10 hours of food when you feel more comfortable. Try different things to see what works best for you. Don't give up until you try different aspects.

Weight gain

It's hard to work on an empty stomach to maintain the same weight. Gaining weight during fasting can be discouraging. However, don't take it as a sign that you should simply stop fasting. You just need to edit some aspects of your post. There are many reasons why you can gain weight. Maybe you eat too much, eat too little, or eat too badly. Gaining weight by eating too much is obvious. If you consume many more calories than you burn, you will gain weight. When you fast, you can eat more than necessary for several reasons. You may unknowingly worry about hunger to alleviate this problem and eat a lot more for each meal. It is easy to understand how this fear can lead to overeating.

Instead of eating everything in sight, start paying attention to what you eat and in what quantities. Keep a food diary and record everything you put in your body. Keeping a food diary can surprise you with what we eat. We might think that all we had was a banana, but after checking the newspaper, we see that we have eaten much more than a banana. If you are someone who eats them unconsciously, someone who eats them when you are stressed or bored will want to take a more conscious look at how you eat.

We will discuss awareness later in this chapter. After reviewing the food diary, look for areas that you can improve on. If you find that you only eat large meals, look for ways to limit what you eat. For example, you can replace a half plate with a salad instead of pasta. It will help you feel saturated without consuming so many calories on a plate full of pasta. If you are worried about being hungry, maybe you will first try to eat small portions and then analyze how you feel afterward? Are you hungry, or are you feeling well? If you are hungry, you can increase the amount of protein and fiber in your meals.

Another reason you can gain weight is that you don't eat enough. It sounds contradictory, but it makes perfect sense when you understand the human body. When our body feels that we are not getting enough nutrients, it automatically decides that we must face hunger. It is an evolutionary state in which our body takes this environmental information and does everything possible to save us, even if we are not hungry. Our body begins to accumulate everything we eat, drastically reduces the metabolic rate, and cannibalizes our muscles if that were not enough. In this situation, you will lose weight only when your body starts focusing on several necessary organs. In this case, you will have to worry about weight gain. This is a risk if you limit both fasting and calories, but it can happen if you don't intentionally control calories. It is very important to eat enough, but not too much or too little. A balanced diet is required to enjoy fasting.

Make improvements, and then talk to your dietitian. They can give you clear tips, recipes, and ideas on eating more and getting rid of hunger. If, after all this, you continue to eat very briefly, it is time to stop fasting and consider talking to your doctor. Something else can happen, and the doctor can help you solve it.

The last reason you can gain weight during fasting is the lack of nutrition. We talked about the importance of a balanced diet, but suppose you have decided not to follow this recommendation. If you eat every day and eat foods high in fat and unhealthy calories, you will eat too many nutrients. Increase fat, which is a natural reaction to excess nutrients. Again, if you plan on eating healthy, try keeping a food diary. To be honest, we all think we are eating healthy, but a food diary can show us exactly where we are not. When you use the diary to analyze meals and make improvements, you will get many benefits. At the end of the day, if you eat healthy, well-balanced meals, and continue gaining weight, talk to a dietitian and doctor. You may have other things in your body, and your doctor/dietician can help you solve the mystery.

CHAPTER 5 - MOTIVATION & HEALTHY HABITS

HOW TO FIND AND NOT LOSE MOTIVATION

The first two weeks of intermittent fasting can be difficult, but sometimes they can be a little disappointing if you don't see your hard work's tangible results. It can almost prevent someone from being motivated, especially if they notice a downsizing in these uncomfortable first few weeks.

Find the fast friend:

It is easier to continue when you know someone is fasting with you. It can be your husband, your relative, or your best friend.

Sit with them and guide them through the basics of your intermittent fasting technique. They are used as support these days when one of you does not want to fast or train. It will be more fun when you have someone with whom you can plan meals, buy food, train, and learn.

Set achievable goals:

It is best to start with goals in the short term that you know you can achieve. When you reach this goal, reward yourself, but don't do it with junk food. It helps to increase your momentum and motivation.

Follow the progress:

It is a great way to see the positive changes that have occurred, following the publication's principle. Take a diary and start writing how you feel and all the progress you are making. It is essential to take the time to see how the body and life change. See how your clothes fit and energy, how you have to play with children, and how your sleep has improved. Be a witness to the progress and make a positive day every time.

You can't hit:

Yes, there are days when you fail and give in to temptation. Be compassionate with yourself. Don't start talking negatively about yourself just because you haven't done the right thing.

Pray and meditate:

When you start feeling discouraged, take time to feed and strengthen your soul and spirit. Pray, read the scriptures, and meditate. This will help you to love yourself despite the challenges in your life.

Focus on the good:

I bet you found more energy in the first few weeks, more preparation, euphoria, and even creativity. It was fantastic, wasn't it? You've probably also had more time available recently, especially if you skip a meal that generally takes "preparation time." What allows you to do this extra time? Think about the extra time you spend with your family or loved ones, all the additional things you do, and how it helps you feel motivated at work when you don't see the expected quick results. Usually, after three or four weeks, the fat loss begins and is fairly stable by that time.

Slow down:

Changes have the time, and it doesn't happen overnight. If you want to lose weight and make sure you stay away, you should lose weight slowly. You can starve and lose a few pounds, but they will not help you. The more gradual and permanent, the simpler weight loss is to maintain. Intermittent fasting is an excellent dietary option and is balanced. Make sure you go slowly. There is no hurry, and you don't have to jump directly.

Be your trainer:

You are the best person to motivate yourself. You can program your mind to think about what you want it to believe. You must behave positively by strengthening your efforts and remembering your motivations. You can program your mind and body every day to become an extraordinary fat-burning machine.

Prepare to forgive yourself:

Don't forget that intermittent fasting is not a walk in the park. You will realize that it is not as easy as people think. You can join a birthday party and, in the meantime, enjoy a delicious meal instead of following a quick schedule. OK, Remember, don't be discouraged because it's normal and you're just human. Instead of punishing yourself, be aware of the mistake, immediately take the road and go above and beyond.

Failures are common:

Temptation can strike, and there will be times when you can give in to your temptations. After all, you're just human. Good, it's a disappointment, but do not think it is a failure.

Be patient:

One of the important obstacles to your diet is the weight loss plateau. You can eat well and exercise properly, but the numbers on the scale don't seem to change. Stairs appear to be blocked for some reason. Well, this is known as a weight loss plateau and is something that every diet has to face. Turn around and congratulate yourself on your success so far. It is part of this weight loss process.

Stay together:

The diet requires some effort, and sometimes it may not seem fun. So don't forget to take care of yourself after reaching your goal. The goal can be large or small. When you reach your destination, your prize doesn't have to be extravagant. Maybe you can buy the nail polish bottle you want! The rewards you display should never be associated with food. Don't reward yourself with a pint of ice cream for losing 5 pounds in ten days. It makes no sense and makes a diet superfluous. When you celebrate your success, you will feel better about yourself and your body. Besides, it will provide you with the motivation needed to continue.

CHAPTER 6 - SET YOUR GOALS AND DO A PRODUCTIVITY PLAN

THE FIRST STEP: CREATE A PLAN.

Concerning intermittent fasting, it may seem daunting. This protocol is useful if you want to check your eating habits and lose weight. However, the annoyance remains the same when it comes to starting with something new. Don't leave. Before you get started, you already know it's not just a diet or some other program, but a lifestyle with specific goals that you want to achieve on time. If you accept this fact, it motivates you to continue. As in any culture, food is an important part of our life. Many of our lives seem to revolve around this business. Therefore, opting for intermittent fasting will change your lifestyle, but you can adapt it to your life. Don't let intermittent fasting decide your life.

Step 1: Choosing a fasting method that is right for you

Depending on your lifestyle, personality, and goals, you can choose the fasting mode or adapt it to your needs. The feeding window should be from 10 to 16. If you are an early riser, you like to train in the morning, and you have to eat something in the morning or after training, 8/16 is the easiest way to start because it is close to today's normal schedule. I recommend trying the 18/6 protocol below if you don't get the desired results.

Assuming 18/6 works for you, but you want to be more aggressive, you can try Eat Stop Eat (also known as One Meal a Day or OMAD) one day a week. Over time, you can increase your frequency based on the results shown. Do not pass the OMAD protocol for prolonged fasting without consulting your doctor first, especially if you take medications for specific health problems. Over time, the doctor may change or stop certain medications.

Step 2: research, research, and more research

A lot of research will be needed to find one approach and the other. Review the information in this book and determine if your priorities and needs align with one of these methods. The main thing is to choose a method that works for you. Your research depends on your goals. Before you get started, define your goals precisely. If you want to change your body's composition, increase muscle mass, and reduce body fat, you must try the 16/8 or 18/6 method. If you are looking for aging and disease prevention, you can consider prolonged fasting 24 hours once or twice a week. Several Facebook groups may be of interest to post and often ask more frequently asked questions. It is equally important to experiment and learn from others so that you are not alone. Usually, these are "closed" groups, so you need to request access.

Step 3: Know the tools you need

Several online applications will make your life easier. There are paid and free applications that will help you make a speed monitor. Intermittent on an empty stomach is a trial and error method. To get started, you can try the following applications:

- Zero
- Fast body
- Fast habit
- My fast
- Follow your post

You won't know what will work for you if you don't try it yourself. These apps will help you keep track of your feeding times, as well as counting calories. You can also follow a diary to track your progress. It helps if you have strong evidence of the intermittent fasting working method or if some of them don't do the job.

Step 4: It begins with a transition time

When you fast, you don't eat. Simple enough, but if you're not used to fasting, you won't be able to spend long periods without eating. You should slowly condition your body so that the transition to fasting methods is smooth. It is no different when something new starts, for example, an exercise program. To get started, you can begin reducing the sugars and carbohydrates processed by your diet.

Step 5: Find the Support

It would help if you had your family and friends. Having a support system helps. Starting this program with a partner will be very helpful. It can be your friend, spouse, or even a relative. You can follow them.

Anyone can use the other as a coach and as moral support. They can fast together and practice together. Whenever you feel like giving up, someone else will motivate you and ensure you stay on the right track.

Step 6: Initially reduce your training tone.

Often, power requires minimalism. Like the resistance of coffee or any alcoholic beverage that distracts when diluted with water, training effectiveness during intermittent fasting can simulate if you also train. But what do we mean by overtraining in this context? The most important examples are exercises of very high intensity for long periods. When you also make your efforts and change your body works, it will burn, and you may end up in pain or not feeling well afterward.

Do not opt for high intensity during the initial phases of the program on an empty stomach. You can gradually increase it. The body needs to get used to regulating the carbohydrates that burn from stored fat use, thanks to the consumption of thermal energy, which can take several weeks. Give yourself some time.

What does the correct intensity mean? In general, you feel very uncomfortable (dizzy, exhausted, and weakened; or suffer from prolonged muscle pain) during or after exercise. An easy way to determine if you are exercising at moderate intensity is through a conversation test. If you can start a normal conversation during the workout (albeit with some difficulty), this is moderate. If you can talk the same or barely breathe with the words, you are under training (low intensity) or higher (high intensity), respectively.

Step 7: Focus on Delayed Satisfaction and Goals

Delayed satisfaction is a useful technique. It works exceptionally well for intermittent fasting. If your colleagues are hungry, your mind will make you give up.

Focus on "why" makes the intermittent fasting (to improve health and lose weight) help you overcome this temptation temporarily. Stay busy not to think about hunger pains, or you keep eating.

Step 8: The priority in choosing a diet high in carbohydrates and proteins.

Be sure to have a meal with complex carbohydrates rich in nutrients before running the satiety mechanism, followed by protein and healthy fats. You can start with a green leafy vegetable salad after the first meat and perhaps avocado for its healthy fats. This will help you plan meals and make sure you have enough protein and carbohydrates. Your eating habits will be better without any extra effort.

Step 9: Take photos of "before" and "work in progress."

Before starting an intermittent fasting protocol, take a photo of yourself. This is a photo of the "first" to see why you decided to follow the path first quickly and how much progress you are making. It will also help you understand the importance of starting now and putting things off for later. After starting, you will find the motivation to overcome all the obstacles encountered. You can measure your progress by comparing it with this image. It will surely make you want to move forward. I admit I hesitated to take pictures" before "because I was embarrassed by my body's appearance. As I wonder, this motivates me to continue reaching my goals.

CHAPTER 7 – IF & LIFESTYLE

To start, all you need is an idea meant for your daily routine, because every day is not so sure. Think again and see when you plan to eat most of the food on an average day. So pay attention to the time you plan to sleep longer. Finally, write down other facts that are essential to your daily routine.

I noticed some important dates and that I initially considered were happy hours with my spouse, friends, and the family dinner, where we have dinner together every day. On average, I decided that my meal hours last from 10:00 to 20:00 from Monday to Friday and from 12:00 to 24:00 on the weekends because I have a fantastic social life. I slept with terrible sleep habits around midnight; I woke up at 8:00 on weekdays and from 2:00 to 12:00 at the latest on the weekends.

Check your notes and select the first 8 hours of the day to view them as a feeding window. Using this program, I would say that a good startup window will be every day from 12:00 to 20:00. In this quick window, it will start automatically every day at 20:00 and quickly until noon. Some people eat three meals in 8 hours, but it is impossible for me, so I eat two moderate portions in portions and as snacks at other times during a meal. You can decide how many meals and snacks to eat during fasting, but you can stay consistent.

Meal planning

Meal planning, also known as meal preparation, involves preparing some or all meals/snacks in advance so you can have them on hand when needed. Preparing meals saves time, so don't prepare meals/snacks every day, and don't start thinking about what you will eat every. When preparing food, there is less room for failure, especially for beginners. The advantage of planning meals is to prepare healthier foods during the feeding period instead of quickly selecting complex and packaged options, which is convenient.

For me, there are many steps to planning meals. Meal planning involves creating complete meals (including recipes), creating a complete shopping list, checking the kitchen to see what you already have and what you need, then editing the shopping list, and finally going shopping. Creating meals requires creativity. Thanks to the global network, there are many recipes and meal ideas for the options available. Being creative doesn't always mean eating the same day after day. Change options for breakfast, lunch, dinner, and snacks.

Season the food differently. Decorate it differently. Let it be soup or salad instead of a saucepan. Make some vegetables. Find ways to increase your protein intake. Add more green leaves to the protein shakes and/or more vegetables or fruit. Choose 2-3 options for lunch, dinner, and snacks. Once you have decided which food you have created and which recipes you have, you should look in the kitchen cabinets, the freezer, the pantry, and the refrigerator to see what you have already eaten, and you do not have to take when buying food. This includes everything; meat, additives, fresh vegetables, fruit fresh, drinks, snacks, spices, herbs, oils, bread, packaging, and more. Check the shopping list to include what you need. Go to the grocery stores and collect the items from the list. Preparing meals consists of taking all the food and cutting everything that needs to be cut, washing everything that needs to be cleaned, pickling everything that requires pickling, and seasoning everything you need.

Taste and cook everything you need to make a backup; cook everything you need to cook, measure everything that needs to be measured in the right portion, and put everything in separate food containers for easy pickup and transfer, if necessary. However, although highly recommended, meal planning and preparation are not required for intermittent fasting.

Portion control, food labels, and measurements

However, portion control is unnecessary when taking an intermittent fast, as no food group is limited and you can technically eat what you want while eating; portion control becomes even more important than preparing meals, but it can also help speed up weight loss with the same such treatment.

For better starts in food preparation, measure food and compress it in containers before storage for later. Another tip to make sure you eat well is to drink a glass of water to make sure you're hungry, and not just thirsty, and make sure you don't overeat. Food labels show the nutritional content/nutritional information, calories, and portion sizes of packaged food. Reading food labels ensures you don't go right away; it's the best portion control. The first thing to check is the portion size. The portion size is usually indicated simultaneously. The number of calories shows the number of calories in a serving. Food labels also contain total fat, cholesterol, sodium, and total carbohydrates per serving. Also, the value of daily % shows how many portions will be counted for your daily consumption; try not to exceed 100% in any category. To succeed during intermittent fasting, it is unnecessary to read and understand food labels, but it can improve results. Net carbohydrate counting is another great topic of discussion about gravity. To count net carbohydrates, subtract dietary fiber from all carbohydrates, which is equal to net carbohydrates. Net carbohydrate counting is only an acceptable way of eating and planning meals, BUT it is not necessary to count net carbohydrates with periodic fasting. The net carbohydrate and calorie counter are NOT required for intermittent fasting. Measurement of food is not necessarily required if intermittent fasting is performed, but it ensures that you do not eat too much. Well, in smaller containers, make sure you eat a large amount of food to be full but not stuffed. Never eat a packet of snacks and reduce distraction while eating, because people usually eat too much during activities like watching TV. Measuring food is important for portion control, but it is not necessary for intermittent fasting.

THE MAINTENANCE OF PSYCHOPHYSICAL WELL-BEING

After an intermittent fasting mode, you are not limited to any food group and can choose food options, BUT your food options remain (as always) valid. It is important to have good nutrition that emphasizes a diet, providing a complete source of minerals, vitamins, and nutrients for the body to function healthier. The diet is considered the sum of all the foods consumed but refers to a specific nutritional intake. On an empty stomach, I try to eat more protein and protein lean that is non-starchy. Choose whole grains and stay away from refined cereals and flour. The fruit will be the best option to preserve the sweets, especially for beginners. Choose products other than dairy products and eat fats and oils in moderation as you choose healthier forms of fats and oils. Fresh fruit and vegetables are better than frozen and preserved ones, but any vegetable is better than none. Choose the protein pieces, increase your protein intake; add vegetarian sources like soybeans and products. Try the non-dairy options almond, soy, or cashews to reduce milk intake because it is one of the world's major allergens. Other important allergens are eggs, peanuts, and crustaceans.

Create carbohydrate overlays instead of the base of meals. When buying pasta, bread, crackers, and more, always look for all the wheat, which is listed as the first ingredient on the nutrition label. Eat half an avocado at least once a day to increase your intake of healthy fats.

According to the USDA, five main guidelines must be followed to meet your nutritional needs. Follow the pattern of healthy eating for life. The nutritional standard is the intake of liquids and foods and their usual way of eating. Compliance with this first guideline guarantees the adequacy of nutrients, a healthy body system, and a lower risk of invading chronic diseases in the body. The second and fourth tips are to focus on the amount of food and liquids consumed and focus on consuming nutrient-rich foods from all major food groups and the transition from bad choices to good choices. The most important are your decisions. You are an important link that makes the difference; you have control over these guidelines. All people are responsible for compliance with these guidelines. The third factor is to reduce the number of calories that are not derived from nutrient-rich foods, such as sugars at high concentrations of fat sodium and Trans and fat-saturated. According to the USDA, healthy meals are made up of whole fruit, fresh vegetables, dairy products, proteins, whole grains, and oils. The fifth guideline teaches you how to share your knowledge with others; It argues that support is necessary for everyone, and we must support healthy eating habits.

Physical activity

Like meal planning, food measurement, reading food labels, and portion control, exercise is unnecessary, but it is useful for overall results during intermittent fasting. The American Heart Association recommends some form of physical activity for at least 30 minutes a day.

Create a training program. Create a day for the legs, a day for the arms, a day for cardio, a day for total body weight, and more. The program becomes more coherent and responsible. If you are already training, intermittent fasting can only improve your performance. The combination of intermittent fasting and exercise maximizes weight loss and/or weight maintenance.

Mentality

The biggest barrier, if any, will be your mentality. The barrier will be the attitudes and assumptions already established in your head, especially about the relationship you have with food and food consumption. Think about your mind and worry more, so you better take care of yourself. To maintain the intermittent lifestyle, eliminate or ignore all previous hypotheses or attitudes associated with diet/lifestyle changes, bodyweight loss, current habits, current habits plans, and changes in general, as well as others. After launch, try to make the best decisions and discipline yourself to follow your plans constantly. To be successful, you need to think and act differently for optimal results.

Survive longer when hungry

Hunger is uncomfortable and/or weak due to a lack of food. Hunger can be physical, but at this point, it can only be desire rather than necessity. The body sometimes reacts as if it were hungry, but sometimes we thirst for liquids, not for food, which is why water consumption is crucial to its success if it is longer fasting windows. To get used to longer fasting windows and / or resist food during the fasting window and reach the feeding window, you need to stay productive. Stay busy with all the necessary resources. It's a great idea to train now or engage in work or personal work.

CHAPTER 8 – IF & FITNESS

The first of the most exciting exercises

This chapter will remind us of the exercise's value, and we will consider types of activities that are particularly useful in the intermittent fasting program.

Benefits of Exercise

As long as we can burn more calories than we consume, we will lose weight and reduce body fat. Fasting is one of the best ways to keep your calorie intake low, but the best way to increase it and get all the benefits is to combine it with an exercise program. First of all, for adults (19 to 64 years old) we have a choice: regardless of the chosen path, there must be several sessions per week to work on strength training so that the muscles are in good shape. This will greatly complement your routine because we know it will improve our lean mass.

Also, there should be two and a half hours of moderate aerobic activity (which includes exercises such as cycling or brisk walking) for a week or half of that time for physical exertion. Jogging falls into this category, as do the most competitive tennis games. This minimal activity will help you maintain your weight if your calorie intake is approximately average. It will also support our bodies when we try to improve heart health, organ wellbeing, etc. This will mean weight loss for those who are fasting because our calorie intake will be below average.

Therefore, a short walk on the weekends and every other day of the week will help us lose weight. This is not a big commitment. Two forty-minute trips to the gym will bring us the same benefits. There is one small caveat, however. Although the above exercise patterns will ensure that our minimum health goals are achieved, daily activity is also required. It doesn't have to be serious and can be divided into ten minutes. Some time in gardening, we could say that we work hard in household chores and take the kids to school, which will ensure that we move enough. Let's take a moment to explore the health benefits of even a minimal amount of exercise. Our chances of developing type 2 diabetes are halved and reduce heart disease or stroke risk by over a third. We are more likely to live longer, and some studies indicate that we can cut our chances of cancer by half. Our bones and muscles will serve us better and longer. Mentally, we reduce the risk of depression and dementia by one third. All these advantages are ADDITIONAL to the advantages that we already receive from an interrupted post (see discussions in the previous chapters). It is often said, but it is extremely precise that our life is increasingly sedentary.

One of the best ways to exercise is to adapt them to our daily lives. Walking instead of driving; after waking up, do strengthening exercises. If we go to work, park your car at the end of the parking lot instead of before entering the office. Go to the shop for lunch or a walk during lunch. Exercise releases endorphins and fresh air wake up the brain; It turned out that our afternoon results improved if we exercised mid-day. But exercise and intermittent fasting are not just two things that we can do, which brings us good.

Most modern thinking agrees that there is a relationship between fasting and exercise, which offers additional benefits for all the things we want to achieve through these two activities. The sum of these two values combinations is greater than the individual benefits offered by each of them. This is synergy. In combination with fasting and exercises, 2 + 2 equals 5! We burn more calories; we see better internal cell repair; we see more mental health benefits. This is because modern thinking undermines the old belief that we should not exercise on an empty stomach. When our parents told us that as children; like not swimming in the sea after dinner, they spoke more reasonably than they intended; When it comes to exercise, swimming before lunch would be much better (not because we should probably be worried about kids). Recent studies show that it is best to train on an empty stomach. To summarize this paragraph: if we practice during fasting, the total benefit is greater than the sum of its parts.

THE BEST EXERCISE TO IMPROVE THE BENEFITS OF FASTING

To be a little (but not very) scientific for some time, the rate of fat burning depends on our sympathetic nervous system (SNS). Two things stimulate our SNS: one is exercise, and the other is not to have a stomach full of food. Therefore, when we fast and exercise, we stimulate a combination of pressure to burn fat. But oxidative stress increases, which promotes muscle growth and strength. We can change it even more if we plan our exercises carefully. Fasting days: use them for low-intensity exercises. There are two reasons:

1) If the sugar level drops, dizziness can attack too much exercise,

2) If the body is desperate for something to record for energy production, it can attack muscle mass, something we want to keep. That's why fasting days are ideal for walking, swimming, and jogging.

<u>Days without fasting</u>: therefore, it is logical that we train intensely during the days we have eaten. These are the times when we go to the gym, run long and hard, or do laps in the pool. If weights are part of our training regimen, do it today without fasting. Likewise, if you are looking for high-intensity short sets such as circuit training, use days off. Also, we should eat with this type of training, preferably within thirty minutes after exercising. However, for many people, the joy of intermittent fasting is easy and flexible. For people with severe weight loss or a muscle-building program, the above tips are needed to achieve the expected results. But for most of us who want to be more agile, healthier, and a little lighter on our feet, just remember that every exercise is good for us, regardless of shape.

A post with basic nutritional tips

If you've been to school in the United States, you've heard what a good meal is. We have seen the graphics and the food pyramid, but what does it look like on your plate? How to choose the food that will give us the best energy? We will answer some of these questions in this section.

It has an excellent website called choosemyplate.gov. On this page, you can learn how to divide meals so that they are well balanced. They will also give you meal plans and the appearance of your plate. Each of them can be adapted to their weight, height, gender, etc. So if you want to have a more detailed view of nutritious meals and how they can work for you, check out the website. It is full of resources that can help you choose the right food during fasting. When you eat a balanced meal, you want to eat a lot of fruit and vegetables. This is your fiber. Sp Yam's yellow is an example of what your meals can be. Half of the plate should contain fruit and vegetables. About a third of the dish should contain cereals, preferably whole grains or starchy vegetables. Proteins such as tofu, fish, meat, and cereals should fill the rest of the dish, slightly smaller than a quarter of the pot. Here's what a balanced meal looks like.

CHAPTER 9 – RECIPES

Well balanced ideas for breakfast

Regardless of whether the breakfast is small or plentiful, try mixing protein and fiber after breaking fast. Write about how you feel in your body after eating. This helps to find out what works and what does not. Some people react negatively to taking sugars and carbohydrates in the morning, so watch your reactions to these elements. Here are some breakfast ideas that give you a good mix of fiber and protein.

Hot oatmeal with fruit, nuts, and yogurt: this is the perfect mix of oat fibered fruit, healthy nut fats, and dairy/protein products.

Whole wheat toast and peanut butter/almond butter: eat a portion of fruit. Try a glass of blueberry or apple. Or, if you want to go crazy, cut the bananas and put them in the peanut butter toast.

Cereals integral with a cup of milk: the milk supplies the proteins, and whole grains are your fiber. If you are still hungry, add fruit or nuts to eat with cereals. Remember to read the list of ingredients in the cereal package. Some cereals claim to be "whole grains," but often they are not. Choose the one that will give you good fiber content.

Whole Eggs and Toast: Add a portion of vegetables if you want to make a bigger breakfast. Think of avocados for healthy fats, or try tomatoes and peppers.

Yogurt and muesli: muesli is a carbohydrate and sweet, so be careful. Add berries, chopped almonds, and flax seeds for added nutritional value, along with power link composite fibers (for example, toast, oat flakes, muesli, cereals) with protein (for example, eggs, yogurt, peanut butter, milk). Follow this breakfast pattern that will please you and hold you until your next meal. Whatever you choose for breakfast, make sure you don't get stuck. Therefore, check the portions and eat all the way through, but not too much.

Balanced lunch

This is consistent with the "table" discussed above.

In this part, we will divide the sections and explain some options for each part. So when you prepare dinner, you can choose things from each section. There is so much variety here that it is difficult to limit it to some recipes. After explaining the ingredients, you can choose the right products for you and create many different dishes. Try to provide at least three groups of meals during lunch.

Fruits and vegetables: you can prepare various chopped vegetables or add them to a salad for dinner. You can also add them to the soup and then prepare the vegetables. For salads, try a mix of green leafy vegetables, radishes, half an avocado, tomatoes, grapes, and carrots.

Or add green leaf-like spinach and add beets, carrots, cucumbers, and tomatoes to the salad. If you don't like salads, try fried vegetables like zucchini and mushrooms in soy sauce or broccoli and baked peppers. Both options are excellent for cereals and proteins. If you prefer lunch, which looks more like a small snack group than a full meal, choose two or three raw vegetables and pieces. When people think of such products, they think of carrots, tomatoes, and celery. Any vegetable will work as long as you agree to eat it cold.

Flakes: after preparing the vegetables, add the cereals. If you want a combination of cereals and proteins, try quinoa, barley, or buckwheat. If these aren't things that interest you, get a portion with potatoes or corn. You can even eat a toast or sandwich with whole wheat bread, meat, dairy products, and vegetables. Salted oat flakes are also an option and are delicious with grated bacon, poached egg, and spinach as an appetizer.

Protein: Protein at lunch can be easy to eat, such as minced meat or meat small enough to be eaten without a fork or knife. However, if you want to eat a variety, try salmon steaks, fried beef, roasted chicken breast, or tuna salad. If it's not your meat, try stewed tofu, roasted chickpeas, bean soup, or lentils. Eggs are also a good protein option.

Dairy Products: You can add dairy products to dinner for more flavors. Cheese is always a desirable ingredient in most foods. During lunch, you can also drink a glass of milk or drink half a glass of yogurt to finish your meal. Here are some ideas for a meal:

- Mason salad with green leafy vegetables, greens, quinoa, cheese, and spices.

- Pieces of roasted chicken and baked potatoes, on the side of chopped peppers and tomatoes.

- Baked sweet potatoes with whole beans, cheese, sauce, and corn. A salad can finish this lunch if the potato alone is not enough.

- Spinach Salad with tomatoes, barley, poached eggs, feta cheese and walnuts, and salsa of your choice.

- Open face salad sandwich with whole wheat croutons and salad.

- Bean soup with a mixture of different types of beans, cooked in bone broth or chicken broth. Some vegetables that work with the soup include pumpkin, celery, carrots, garlic, and onion cooked with soup. Barley, egg pasta or rice can also be added to the soup. There is so much variety here.

Find some recipes online that interest you and cook them for lunch. Just remember to give the right proportion of vegetables, fruits, cereals, and proteins. The goal is not a daily lunch. The key tip is to prepare dinners over the weekend, store them in the refrigerator (or freezer) and take them with you on a business day. Make sure your lunch is full and continue until the last meal of the day.

Well balanced ideas for dinner

Dinner is the last meal before fasting. If you run out of windows to eat before bedtime, choose foods that won't wake you up at night. In this situation, stay away from highly salty foods, heavy spices, or high-fat foods. These products disturb sleep. If you have a few hours between your last meal and sleep, don't hesitate to eat things that will give you fullness. Remember that mixing protein and fiber is a key strategy for choosing satiety.

Here and several ideas for meals:

● Wholemeal spaghetti and alb and turkey meatballs with tomato sauce sprinkle with grated Parmesan cheese from several small salads. You can add spinach to tomato sauce.

● Salmon with asparagus, baked tomatoes, and quinoa.

● Chicken curry with brown rice, spinach, and carrots.

● Beans with beans, borlotti beans, and black beans. Serve with wholemeal tortilla, cheese, and chives. Chilies should contain tomatoes and onions, but you can also add peppers, squash, or carrots to fix it.

● Fried tofu with asparagus, peppers, onions, almonds, sesame, and green beans. It can be served with brown rice or barley.

It is a good idea to diversify your meals. Take several meatless meals during the week and add at least two meals with fish. This will provide you with various nutrients and help you not get bored with your menu. Cooking all these meals can be overwhelming if you don't like cooking. If you are interested, you can cook meals on the weekend and store them in the refrigerator or freezer. This will help you plan your meal for the week.

If you want to try something different, you can use one of the meal delivery services that provide full meals or meal ingredients, depending on your nutritional needs. They can be a good option if you don't know how to cook because they will provide everything and provide detailed instructions on how to make your products.

Either way, avoid eating out every day and try to skip easy meals in the freezer unless they are packs of frozen vegetables. Ramen noodles are also not a balanced meal, despite what your roommate taught you in college.

RECIPES

Muffins with broccoli
Ingredients:
- 2 teaspoons of butter, soft
- 2 eggs
- 2 cups of almond flour
- 1 cup of broccoli, chopped
- 1 cup of almond milk
- 1 teaspoon of baking powder

Directions:
1. In a bowl, mix the eggs with flour, broccoli, milk, yeast, and mix very well.
2. Cupcake ingredient: a container with a mixture of ghee divides the broccoli; add it to the oven, and bake at 350 ° C for 30 minutes.
3. Give these muffins for breakfast.

***

Pasta and Salad

Although pasta is not considered the best food option for people who want to lose weight, you can still add a delicious pasta meal to your daily diet and still have a calorie deficit. It is important to pay attention to the amount of pasta and other ingredients contained in food. This pasta with shrimp and salad is a truly delicious meal that you can eat at any time. It has a moderate amount of calories, and each serving provides around 465 calories.

Ingredients:

• Half a cup of dried rigatoni

• Cook according to the instructions on the paste container.

• Half a spoonful of pine nuts

• Three black olives, you can choose large ones and cut them into slices

• Two teaspoons of grated parmesan

• Half a cup of dried tomatoes in the sun, empties the container and then blend in a blender

You will also need additional ingredients to prepare a salad. These include:

• A quarter cup of chopped tomatoes

• Half a spoonful of balsamic vinegar

• A cup of romaine lettuce

• Half a glass of cucumber slices

Directions:

As you can see, it is elementary to prepare a meal and also very fast: just cook the pasta, mix them, prepare the salad and you are ready to eat.

***

Breakfast with pork bagels

Ingredients:

- 1 chopped yellow onion
- one tablespoon of clarified butter
- 2 pounds of ground pork
- Two eggs
- 2/3 cup of tomato sauce
- A pinch of salt and black pepper
- One teaspoon pepper

Directions:

1. Heat a pan with clarified butter over medium heat, add the onions, stir and cook for 3-4 minutes.

2. In a bowl, combine the meat with fried onions, eggs, tomato sauce, salt, pepper, and paprika, mix well and arrange six rolls with your hands.

3. Arrange the bagels with the meat in a lined pan and bake at 400 °F for 40 minutes.

4. Divide the sandwiches into plates and serve them for breakfast.

***

Baked eggs

Ingredients:

• One cup spinach

• 4 ounces chopped bacon

• 2 eggs

Directions:

1. Heat pan over medium heat, add bacon and stir for 4 minutes.

2. Add spinach, salt, and pepper, mix, cook for another 1 minute, remove the heat and divide into four forms.

3. Divide the beaten eggs into each shape, put them in the oven, and cook at 400 ° F for 15 minutes.

4. Serve the eggs in the oven for breakfast.

***

Meatballs with Spaghetti

This meal contains 330 calories per serving. If you increase by three, you will get a meal with a portion of 990 calories.

To prepare a plate of meatballs and spaghetti, you need the following **ingredients**:

• Four spinach leaves

• Sweet potatoes

• A quarter teaspoon of oregano

• Four cups of spelled, cooked

• A spoonful of chopped onion

• Egg white

• Four tsp of turmeric

• A pinch of pepper and salt

• About 115 grams of ground turkey (may seem like a lot, but it's still a low-calorie option)

Preheat the oven before you start. Set the range to about 180 degrees Celsius.

In the steps:

Mix (manually) the ground turkey, the spinach leaves, the proteins, the turmeric, the pepper, the salt, the oregano, the onion spelled, and the onion. After thoroughly mixing the ingredients, manually divide the mixture into four parts, and then roll up each of them. They should be about an inch in diameter.

Cover the pan with parchment and place the balls on the paper, distributing them evenly. Put the pan in the oven and let them cook for about half an hour. Make sure they are golden before removing them. When the meatballs are in the range, wash the sweet potatoes and peel them.

After peeling them, use a potato peeler to make ribbons from a sweet potato. Put these tapes in boiling water with a pinch of salt, and then dry them properly. When the meatballs are ready for cooking, remove them from the oven. Serve the meatballs with strips of sweet potatoes.

***

Baked vegetables with rosemary and Serrano ham

Each serving provides around 322 calories. You will receive approximately 21 g of protein and 10 g of fiber per serving.

Ingredients:

- A spoonful of sherry vinegar
- Two teaspoons of olive oil.
- Two teaspoons of rosemary, fresh and chopped
- About 220 grams of asparagus must be cut into small pieces
- Approximately 220 grams of cabbage of Brussels, so pick one small to mid •
- Two tablespoons of cheese Manchego shaved
- About 30 grams of raw ham; tear the ham into small pieces
- Pepper

Directions:

Turn on the oven at around 220 degrees Celsius.

In a pan, put the asparagus and Brussels sprouts. Sprinkle with oil, rosemary, and a little black pepper. Let it cook in the oven. Remember to mix the vegetable mixture once while it is still in the range after cooking. Add vinegar and ham. Put the pan back in the oven for a minute or two. When serving, sprinkle the Manchego cheese on a plate.

***

Meat and egg

Ingredients:

- one pound of pork, ground
- ¼ beef, ground
- ½ beef, ground
- one tablespoon of maple syrup
- ½ teaspoon of sage, dried
- ½ teaspoon of rosemary, dried
- ½ teaspoon of dried thyme
- two tablespoons of olive oil

Directions:

1. In a bowl, combine the pork with beef, beef liver, maple syrup, sage, rosemary, thyme, salt, and pepper, mix and form 4 pies of this mixture.

2. Heat the pan with half the oil over medium heat, add the meatballs, cook for 5 minutes on each side and divide into plates.

3. Heat the same pan with the rest of the oil, break the eggs, fry them, divide them next to the meatballs, and serve.

***

Pumpkin soup with stewed beef

For many people, a truly balanced meal must contain vegetables and meat. This is excellent because it offers the benefits of both types of food. Here, we get a little creative by introducing some solid meat and vegetable soup onto the plate. It is a very simple meal to prepare and also has few calories. Each serving provides around 450 calories. Let's start with the **ingredients**:

• A cup of shiitake mushrooms; cut them to prepare them.

• About two teaspoons of olive oil.

• About 85 grams of beef fillet. Remember to cut the steak into thin slices. Of course, you can increase the amount of meat added to increase the calories in a meal, making it a great choice for a daily meal.

• 1 onions. Cut the onion into slices

• About half of a Bulgarian cup.

In addition to all the above ingredients, you will also need a pumpkin soup. You can do it yourself, but it will give you more time to prepare dinner. Instead, it is worth buying a pre-cooked butter soup. If you choose this path, try selecting the low sodium option and see if you can find organic pumpkin soup.

To prepare the meat, fry the slices of meat, mushrooms, and onions. Use olive oil to fry these ingredients.

On the site, start with bulgur. From this moment, add the fried meat over the bulgur. Finally, don't forget to serve the walnut soup. Butter soup can be heated before serving.

***

Lemon, dill, and salmon

Below is a low-calorie meal, which is ideal if you want to start the day slowly but wants to choose a meal instead of muesli or other snacks. This is a delicious meal that provides a healthy salmon dose, a species of fish known to be rich in essential fatty acids, such as omega-3 fatty acids. It is good for heart health, for improving cholesterol and for brain health. Part of this dish provides around 261 calories. This means that if you decide to turn it on, you will still have many extra calories you can play with for the rest of the day.

Ingredients:

- A teaspoon of dill
- A spoonful of lemon juice.
- A cup and a half of broccoli
- About 140 grams of salmon, the best type caught in the wild.

Directions:

Chop the broccoli and steam them.

Just add the salmon to a pan and sprinkle with dill and lemon juice. It is best to cook this dish over low heat, around 110 degrees Celsius. Preheat the oven before putting it in the pan. Now, when the oven is hot, add a baking sheet with salmon for about 15 minutes.

***

Pasta Pesto

Next on our list is a delicious pasta dish with just over 400 calories and contains a good mix of meat and vegetables to help you load healthy nutrients. Like other recipes, this can be easily duplicated to increase calorie content and make it the perfect option for celebrating training days.

Ingredients:

• Third-cup chicken breast: cut into small pieces.

• Approximately one-third of a cup of green beans. Boil the beans in advance

• Several cherry tomatoes cut in half

• A cup of linguine - cook even earlier

• About a quarter cup of pesto

• Tart grated Parmesan cheese

• 1 tablespoon of oil

• A pinch of pepper and salt

Directions:

Take a pan and add the sliced chicken breast; cook for 10 minutes with a tablespoon of oil. Add boiled beans, tomatoes, salt, pepper, and pesto sauce. Now add the linguine to your mix.

Finally, sprinkle with Parmesan cheese while serving this meal.

***

Cauliflower Cakes

Ingredients:

- 1 head of cauliflower, separate florets
- 2/3 cup of almond flour
- one tablespoon of yeast
- Two eggs
- one teaspoon of turmeric powder
- two tablespoons of butter
- A pinch of salt and black pepper

Directions:

1. Put the cauliflower flowers in the pot, add water to cover them, cook over medium heat for 8 minutes, strain well, put the cauliflower in the food processor, and blend well.

2. In a bowl, combine the cauliflower with flour, eggs, yeast, salt, pepper, and turmeric, mix well and form medium pancakes with this mixture.

3. Heat the ghee's pan over medium heat, add pancakes, cook for 3 minutes on each side, divide them into plates, and serve breakfast.

***

Quinoa with spicy tofu

Are you looking for something low in calories, ideal for the digestive system, and something else? So try this fantastic quinoa dish served with a little tofu. You just need ingredients, and preparing food is extremely simple. This meal provides around 320 calories per serving.

Ingredients:

• A teaspoon of coriander

• A cup of quinoa - boiled quinoa

• About two tablespoons of avocado cubes

• Three tablespoons of diced pepper

• About 50 grams of tofu; choose one hard and cut them into cubes

• Two teaspoons of lime juice, preferably fresh lime.

There are no special or complicated instructions for preparing this meal. Simply combine all the ingredients listed above, serve, and enjoy.

***

Summer Farrotto

This particular recipe is truly unique if you have to load up after a hard day at the gym.

Ingredients:

- A cup of yellow pumpkin, diced
- Boneless and skinless chicken breasts, about 85 grams
- Sliced red onion
- Half a cup, barley, dry
- A spoonful of grated parmesan
- A spoonful of chopped parsley
- Two tablespoons of olive oil

Directions:

Divided into two parts after collecting all the ingredients, we begin preparing a meal: start using a spoonful of olive oil to brown the chicken in a pan. Add some pepper and salt to the chicken. Cut the chicken into small pieces.

When the oil remains in the pan, add the pumpkin and onion, fry these two ingredients. Add the spelled and make sure it is covered with the previously added oil. Now add about two-thirds of a glass of water to the mixture and let the mixture boil. When the mixture boils, stir once and then reduce the heat of the oven. Cover the mixture with a lid and cook for about 20 minutes. After 20 minutes, add parsley, parmesan, and chicken. Serve and enjoy.

***

Keto sandwich 90 seconds

Ingredients:

• One tablespoon of butter

• three tablespoons of almond flour

• one teaspoon of psyllium powder

• One egg

• A pinch of salt

Directions:

1. Melt the butter in the microwave for 20 seconds (in a pan)

2. Add the psyllium powder, almond flour, baking powder, salt, and eggs on a baking sheet.

3. Mix the ingredients well with a fork

4. Put the plate at high temperature for 90 seconds

5. Remove the bread from the mold and cut it into half to form two pieces of sandwich

6. Make sure that the food is a crispy pan with butter if you take lunches in a more grilled direction

***

Butter coffee

You can choose your favorite cheese.

Ingredients:

- 1 cup of water
- two tablespoons of coffee
- one tablespoon of grass-fed butter
- one tablespoon of coconut oil

Directions:

1. Prepare a cup of coffee to taste. A cup of Turkish coffee is preferred. Boil the ground coffee in water for about five minutes, then strain into a bowl. You can use a Moka pitcher or a French coffee pot.

2. Pour the prepared coffee into the blender, as well as butter and coconut oil. Stir for about ten seconds. You will immediately see that it is light and creamy.

3. Pour the coffee and butter into the cup and enjoy it! Add any ingredient of your choice, such as cinnamon.

***

Bread with pumpkin and spices

Ingredients:

- 2 cups of almond flour
- 1/2 cup of coconut flour
- 1/2 cup of erythritol
- one tablespoon of baking powder
- teaspoons of spices for pumpkin pie
- One pinch of sea salt
- 1 cup of pumpkin puree
- 3/4 cups of melted butter
- 1/3 cup of thick cream
- Four large eggs
- 1/4 cup of chopped walnuts

Directions:

1. Preheat the oven to 350°F and grease the pan.
2. Combine coconut flour, almond flour, sugar-free sweetener, pumpkin spices, yeast dough, salt, and mix well in a bowl.
3. In a food processor, combine pumpkin butter, thick cream, and eggs and mix gently. Beat the wet ingredients in a dry mix, then fold the walnuts.
4. Pour the mixture into the pan and cook for 55 to 65 minutes until the knife inserted in the medium comes out clean.
5. Switch off the oven and let the bread cool for 15 minutes.
6. Remove the loaf and put it on a grill to cook thoroughly. Then cut into 12 slices.

CONCLUSION

The 16/8 intermittent fasting diet is counted among the most popular dietary regimens of the moment. It is easy to follow, economically sustainable, allows you to lose weight quickly, and helps keep sugar under control.

Regarding the hours dedicated to food consumption, it is crucial to emphasize the importance of bringing to the table balanced meals, characterized by whole grains and good fats (coming from sources such as extra virgin olive oil and avocado), proteins with high biological value.

Famous worldwide also thanks to VIPs such as Jennifer Aniston - who declared during an interview that she has been following it for some time - the 16/8 intermittent fasting diet has been the focus of scientific attention several times.

Among the studies that can be called out is this 2014 paper, which involved teams of experts active in various departments at the

University of Illinois at Chicago.[3]

This review study - the results of which need further investigation - found that intermittent fasting may prove more effective than simple caloric restriction to control blood sugar and reduce the risk of type 2 diabetes in overweight or obese BMI individuals.

When talking about intermittent fasting diet 16/8, it is essential to mention also side effects. Among these stands out that, in many cases, those who decide to follow the regime tend to exaggerate the caloric intake in the hours dedicated to food consumption (with not very positive consequences on weight).

Not to be neglected is also the frequent occurrence of side effects such as a strong sense of weakness. For example, in light of this aspect and other circumstances, if looking for a pregnancy, a situation not compatible with intermittent fasting. Before starting whatever diet, I always recommend asking for advice from one's doctor.

Thank you for purchasing this book. I hope it helps you achieve your goals quickly. Very few people decide to change and improve themselves.

Before we say goodbye, I'd like you to pay attention to one detail that ran through the entire book. What makes a difference is DOING. This is what will make your health and your body better. So, resolve to commit every day until you reach your goal.

Our short journey is coming to an end, but this is where your new journey begins: loving yourself and taking care of yourself. Here's to

---

[3] https://pubmed.ncbi.nlm.nih.gov/24993615/

your success!

SOURCES

The Obesity Code, by Jason Fung, MD (Greystone Books, 2016)

Metabolic Effects of Intermittent Fasting - *Annual Review of Nutrition*, August 2017.

Effects of intermittent fasting on health, aging, and disease - de Cabo R, Mattonson MP. *New England Journal of Medicine*, December 2019.

Effect of Alternate-Day Fasting on Weight Loss, Weight Maintenance, and Cardioprotection Among Metabolically Healthy Obese Adults: A Randomized Clinical Trial - *JAMA Internal Medicine*, May 2017.

Alternate-day fasting in nonobese subjects: effects on body weight, body composition, and energy metabolism - *American Journal of Clinical Nutrition*, January 2005

Alternate-day fasting in nonobese subjects: effects on body weight, body composition, and energy metabolism - *American Journal of Clinical Nutrition*, January 2005

www.ingramcontent.com/pod-product-compliance
Lightning Source LLC
Chambersburg PA
CBHW050744030426
42336CB00012B/1652